The Covid Safety Handbook

Staying Safe In An Unsafe World

Violet Blue

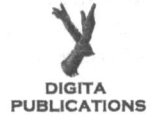

DIGITA
PUBLICATIONS

Copyright © 2024 by Violet Blue. Violet Blue® is a registered trademark. All rights reserved.

This book may not be reproduced, in whole or part, in any form (beyond that copying permitted by Sections 107 and 108 of U.S. Copyright Law and except by reviewers for the public press), without written permission from the publisher.

ISBN: 979-8-9916973-0-9 (ebook)

ISBN: 979-8-9916973-1-6 (paperback)

ISBN: 979-8-9916973-2-3 (audiobook)

Cover design: Violet Blue®, violetblue.com. N95 mask respirator element use under Creative Commons Zero license (CC0 1.0 Universal), Wikimedia Commons, 2023. N95 cup mask element under iStock Standard License, credit: Vladayoung. Flat-fold respirator mask element under iStock Standard License, credit: Gohan.

Title fonts: "Coolvetica" use is Larabie Fonts Freeware Fonts freeware for personal and commercial purposes; "Ronaldson Gothic CAT" use under SIL Open Font License, Version 1.1, credit to Peter Wiegel (catfonts.de). Interior art: N95 mask respirator element use under Creative Commons Zero license (CC0 1.0 Universal), Wikimedia Commons, 2023.

Editing services by Thomas S. Roche, Sarah Clark.

Audiobook narration services provided by: Keira Grace, kiraomans.com.

Published in the United States by Digita Publications, Digitapub.com, inquiries to sales@digitapub.com (U.S.).

DEDICATION

THIS BOOK IS DEDICATED to:
- Tinu
- Russ Kick
- Gary Floyd
- Luis Magdaleno
- Justin du Coeur
- John Erhardt
- Kit Golan
- Richard Stringfellow
- Euterpe Jones
- Jane Greenawalt
- Mindy Lym
- Jamie Emerson
- Skye P
- Joseph C
- Erez Morag
- For Disability Justice

Adrienne Ballerine
Beverly Bush
Dave and Smudge
David Strauss; Brad W.S.
Barb Moermond
Irene Duncan
June Muoi Huynh, @thelonghaul_covidjourney
John Robert Blair
Jacques Frechet and Briana Cavanaugh
Frank Parnell Corcoran, Jr.
Jan Z.
and
In memory of Thomas Lord

TABLE OF CONTENTS

INTRODUCTION	VII
1. WHY WE STAY SAFE	1
2. TRUST THE TOOLS	19
3. PLAN IT, JANET	41
4. COVID BOUNDARIES	59
5. TALKING ABOUT COVID	74
6. COVID GASLIGHTING	93
7. LONG COVID AND RELATIONSHIPS	112
8. COVID PERSONALITY CHANGES	128
9. ISOLATION AND CONNECTION	141
10. MAKE ANGER USEFUL	151
11. REFERENCES AND RESOURCES	169

12.	SURVEY RESPONSES	195
13.	ACKNOWLEDGEMENTS	207
14.	ABOUT THE AUTHOR	210

INTRODUCTION
STAND TOGETHER

I HAD BEEN SHIVERING in a muddy tent on camera for five hours gripping a microphone and manipulating volunteers for various international aid organizations into telling me where the bodies were being kept when we finally got a break from the din of nonstop gunfire. One hour earlier, two trainees had run past us toward one of the roads, terrified, fleeing the site altogether. I kept the interview rolling.

It was 2012: my first year as a session leader for UCSF's Complex Humanitarian Emergency Training (CHE Leadership Training).[1] This took place in a sprawling forest campsite at Anthony Chabot Regional Park, Oakland, California (not far from the Chabot Gun Club's outdoor shooting range). CHE Leadership Training was a fully immersive on-site simulation, an overnighter that began at dawn and was based on the Libyan-Tunisian crisis. Trainees and session leaders represented Médecins Sans Frontières, The UN World Food

Programme, The International Federation of Red Cross, and the International Medical Corps.

The CHE began with trainees entering the simulation upon arrival. They were greeted by "military" and processed, or isolated and detained, before each team was called into one of five sessions: Wilderness Medicine (wound triage), Geneva Conventions Training (mock abduction and interrogation), Water Training (refugee camp water systems), and Interacting with the Media. The fleeing pair who'd sped by my training had come from the Geneva Conventions session, and did not return. A Médecins Sans Frontières colleague remarked, "If they can't deal with what happens to us, they can't do this work. Better to know now."

I was drawn to lead the CHE sessions after growing up at the end of the HIV/AIDS crisis in San Francisco's queer Castro district and fully understanding, firsthand, how the role of media distorted public understanding of health and science, prolonged the crisis and suffering, and added to the body count. Essential to my survival and getting me off the streets was becoming part of SF's harm reduction movement: participating in public health outreach, science and prevention education, and turning fear and misinformation about HIV into community-appropriate prevention strategies (and getting people tested). I was also drawn to be part of the CHE's work in 2012 because I was working with colleagues in New York at *CBS News*, journalists who had been on the ground during 9/11 and still seethed about media coverage and mischaracterizations of first responders in the aftermath of the disaster.

My job was to portray a sensationalist reporter visiting the refugee camp, remain in character, and put volunteers on the spot to learn how to deal with misinformation traps and representation under pressure.

My CHE sessions were popular and highly regarded for their accuracy in replicating what relief workers encountered in the field.

I was invited by Dr. John Zeigler to lead a media training in a summer course called "Emerging Topics in Global Health" for the UCSF Global Health Masters Program. Its focus was the public understanding of science in general, and in particular how scientists communicate effectively with the media, particularly around public health crisis communication.

This training was in a classroom: I got to forgo the CHE's gunshots, bug bites, atmospheric drama of lurking actors, and sticky fake blood. Dr. Ziegler began with remarks about the public understanding of science and critical role of the media in health messages. Next, I explained how the media looks at health "stories" and how important it is to frame messages for a lay audience, structured around avoiding misrepresentation or distortion of facts. Then we got to the fun stuff: the hands-on bits.

The class was presented with a crisis and split into two teams. Our crisis setting was based on one that actually occurred in Ghana, where rumors, spread by the media, almost derailed a massive public health campaign.[2]

In 2007, Ghana held a national health programme where it administered deworming tablets to schoolchildren, jointly organized by the Ghana Health Service, the Ghana Education Service, and UNICEF. Within hours of the start, rumors circulated and became unsubstantiated reports on local radio stations about childrens' deaths and serious side effects. People panicked. Traffic was jammed, parents rushed their kids to hospitals by the hundreds, and in some instances, teachers were attacked and schools were shut. Trust in public health was broken and a safe prevention tool (in that situation, a deworming tablet) was believed to be of worse consequences than the outcome of infection. Sound familiar?

The UCSF Global Health Masters Program students came back with great plans. Their plans included unifying community-based outreach in conjunction with local leadership (like teachers). Taking parents' concerns seriously and transparently investigating the rumors. Creating a clear messaging plan that communicated the harms and consequences of infection, and the science of prevention. And critically, for my part, communicating all of this to the media in ways that won't get misinterpreted. This is what actually happened to turn the crisis around in Ghana; some of the students noted it was far from the many, many horrific public health decisions during the HIV/AIDS crisis. Covid-19 arrived seven years later, and I often wonder what those students have done since.

The many parallels between the HIV/AIDS crisis and ongoing Covid-19 pandemic are undeniable. The queer San Francisco neighborhood I grew up in was a ghost town from the virus's toll when I became homeless at thirteen. I never knew the bustling, populated, joyous Castro that existed before the AIDS crisis (although police harassment and abuse of residents remained the same).

On March 5 2020, San Francisco announced its first local cases of the novel coronavirus,[3] then was the earliest and strictest city in the US to enact a shelter in place order,[4] and—for a brief moment—was united in community care and held the title of most lives saved in the US by our actions.[5] We knew it was because we had done this before as a city, saving each other during the AIDS crisis and abandonment to that virus by the US federal government and US CDC (Centers for Disease Control and Prevention).

Then, the city of San Francisco reversed course and began a cycle of mass Covid infection that would see my hometown continually have the highest wastewater readings and cases in the state of California since the virus evolved into Omicron. I watched my beloved Castro neighborhood sickened by Covid waves on repeat. I watched friends working retail in my local shops unable to finish sentences as they struggled with Long Covid after their second and third infections. I witnessed so many of the infected and reinfected, my friends and neighbors, some who were survivors of the AIDS crisis, just... disappear from daily life. All while the US CDC urged people to wash their hands and insisted Covid is just a "high risk" person problem, media ignored Covid-19 just as it had with HIV/AIDS, and pundits mocked prevention or branded communications about Covid's dangers and unknowns as "hysterical."

One thing Dr. John Zeigler said during our Ghana exercise with UCSF's Global Health Masters' students stayed with me from the beginning of Covid-19 and rings louder in my head every week as the pandemic continues. He said: "The pathway from evidence to sound policy often relies on the public understanding of science, and the mass media is the main messenger." To prevent disaster, he believed, it was critical to translate science and health outcomes for a lay audience. That's why *The Covid Safety Handbook* is designed for lay people as well as a book you can consult for resources, ideas, and pandemic wayfinding tips.

Covid is a global pandemic and no one nation can declare it "over." Yet the world seems to be stuck with a US CDC-led response to Covid-19. This is despite the fact that in 2022 when the US passed one million deaths it began to "unwind" its Covid response, and America was ranked third-worst in *Think Global Health*'s High-Income Countries on Cumulative Reported Covid-19 Mortality.[6] The following year, 2023, the United States held 4% of the world's population and 16% of global Covid-19 deaths.[7] And we know the mass disabling event of Long Covid will only amplify the scope of America's ongoing Covid-19 disaster. Long Covid has never been a metric of the pandemic. But it *must* be. It's more important than ever to understand that the US CDC represents a complete misunderstanding of public health and social contracts.

This book was begun and finished in Aotearoa New Zealand, where I am currently in Wellington researching and writing a book about New Zealand's Covid-19 response in the pandemic's first three years. Typically, a country's "pandemic success" regarding Covid-19 is ranked by deaths per capita. Aotearoa is globally lauded as saving the most lives of any other country. In 2023, Aotearoa attained Bloomberg's title of having the lowest Covid-19 deaths among wealthy nations.[8] Bloomberg also rated New Zealand at the top of its Covid resilience ranking among 10 metrics including case counts, deaths, testing capabilities, vaccine supply agreement, health care system capacity, impact of restrictions on the economy, and citizens' freedom of movement.[9] That year, New Zealand counted 3,250 total lives lost to Covid.[10]

If Aotearoa had used the same response as the United States, it would have translated to a death toll easily six times as many deaths (1 9,900).[11] But we can't hope to understand Aotearoa's Covid successes by counting its losses–or by editing out the principal role of community, and Indigenous cultures and values, from history's record.

When I was a homeless kid in San Francisco long after it had been abandoned by the federal government to HIV/AIDS, my neighborhood was equally a place where I watched friends die from the disease as well as a place of community care, resilience, organizing to save one another, and fighting back against anti-science steeped in stigma. The care circles that formed to sneak magazines into hospitals for AIDS patients, hand out flyers about safer sex, and deliver food to homebound patients also formed to give us street kids food, places to go on holidays, ways to form job skills, and the resilience of chosen family (our values).

Remember in the beginning of the pandemic when everyone came together to help each other stay safe, do prevention, care for one another, make too much bread for each other, and flash each other "V for victory" signs when we hit prevention milestones together? We are still here.

The Covid Safety Handbook is informed by the global, national, local, and neighborhood care circles coming together under the banner of Covid prevention to center science, accurate and non-judgemental information, inclusiveness, and equity in public health. This book draws strength from all the tireless variant hunters and wastewater trackers around the world who struggle to maintain and share the work of Covid-19 surveillance. It is inspired by the global formations of community-led mask blocs, Corsi-Rosenthal Box workshops, Covid-safe maps and meetup networks, Covid safety subreddits (and Discords, Facebook groups, and Slacks), clean air in schools organizations around the world, and those fighting to reinstate masks in healthcare everywhere.

This is a handbook shaped by the oracles of disability activism and disability justice. This book is indebted to the fight against medical racism. This book is humbled and informed by the people with Long Covid, the LC communities, and the massive global movement of Long Covid networks who refuse to give up, who keep organizing and sharing information, fighting for prevention, recognition, and help, who refuse to be silent or left behind. This book is in solidarity with the journalists out there who see all of this and know the Covid-19 pandemic is far from over.

All of these groups comprise a global phenomenon that formed only within the past few years and is growing, undeniable in its increasing strength and momentum.

This book is made possible by Kickstarter backers, patrons, everyone who answered survey questions, each person who said a kind word to someone struggling in our comments or chat, everyone who commented, messaged, and emailed; everyone who did test reads, psychology reads, and sensitivity reads. It's the product of years of weekly Pandemic Roundups, a newsletter and community that has shared news, information, and support every single week of this ongoing pandemic. It's comprised of voices I'm honored to feature, many of my own pandemic heroes, including Yaneer Bar-Yam, Dianna Corwin, Dr. Cat Hicks, Tithi Bhattacharya, Dr. George Taleporos, Julia Doubleday, and many more.

Stay apart, stand together, mask up, and stay strong.

Violet Blue

Wellington, Aotearoa New Zealand

2024

WHY WE STAY SAFE

> *"If there was one thing that I would not have predicted—but, arguably, should have been able to predict—regarding the Covid-19 pandemic, it's the degree to which my fellow academics, particularly physicians and scientists, would contribute to public fear, misunderstanding, and doubt about public health interventions utilized to mitigate the worst of the pandemic."*
> —Dr. David H. Gorski, Science-Based Medicine

ONE THING NEARLY EVERYONE on this planet shares is a powerful sense memory of how *quiet* it was in March 2020. The stillness was overwhelming. No one of any generation had ever heard the world like that, and probably never will again. The quiet seemed to amplify everything we felt, from fear and hyper-vigilance to hope and connection, and more.

We stayed put because a new virus came out of nowhere and rapidly infected and killed people. Covid-19 (SARS-CoV-2) had learned how to jump from person to person with a swift and lethal ferocity. It was terrible, those reports of people drowning alone in their own lung fluid while doctors and nurses could barely do more than watch.

We didn't know how people were catching it. Medical professionals didn't know how to treat it or save people. People in major cities couldn't sleep due to the sounds of refrigerated trucks running all night.[1] Hospitals and morgues ran out of room for all the dead bodies.[2] Many healthcare workers died.[3] Many others would develop Long Covid.[4] In the United States, many of us sheltered in our homes and clapped for them at dusk. They couldn't hear us. But we had to do *something*.

In March 2020 around 75% of the United States came together to stay put under unevenly implemented "shelter in place," "safer at home," and "stay at home" orders.[5] In other countries, people stayed put under actual lockdowns with testing, tracing, and quarantine programs. This was to give science some runway to hopefully develop vaccines and treatments, to learn how to mitigate spread, to slow the virus down from ripping through populations, and so officials—we were all told—could plan and place mitigations in place for safe re-opening of society.

In 2020 the World Health Organization and United States Centers for Disease Control and Prevention both assured the public Covid-19 was not airborne, that it jumped person to person through droplets from coughs and sneezes and from surfaces.[6] Society re-opened with incorrect prevention guidance about droplets, although mitigations like masks were in place for a short time. Vaccination rolled out in phases and was made a substitute for prevention in 2021.

But Covid-19 was airborne. Many knew this in 2020.[7] By 2022, data journalist Farah Hancock and University of Auckland aerosol chemist Dr Joel Rindelaub teamed up for a Covid-prevention guide educating Aotearoa New Zealand citizens on how to use CO_2 (Carbon Dioxide) readings to avoid airborne transmission.[8] New Zealand would later be hailed as a global success story in saving lives and protecting its population and diverse communities from Covid.

It would take years for the WHO and US CDC to formally communicate information connecting Covid with airborne transmission to the public—mostly through random social media posts. In April 2024, the WHO issued a report finally acknowledging Covid-19 requires public infection control for airborne transmission.[9] The CDC disregarded the WHO's report, upholding guidance for droplet transmission, only acknowledging in August 2024 Covid's airborne transmission in social media posts about clean air, avoiding the fact entirely in its updated Covid prevention guidance published online.[10]

The White House in July 2021 told Americans not to mask if they were vaccinated.[11] Shorty after, the US experienced its largest and deadliest surge due to the Omicron variant, which had evolved through unmitigated spread to transmit faster and essentially diminish the first vaccines, which were calibrated for a much different, older strain of the virus. This began a cycle of repeated mass infections in a futile quest for "herd immunity." We were told that our high vaccination rate would solely protect us.

Horrifically, we were also told that only "at risk" people needed to worry now, sacrificing the lives of disabled, chronically ill, immunocompromised, and elderly while creating conditions in which these populations are essentially sentenced to solitary confinement if they want to survive.[12] A 2022 University of Georgia study found that white Americans cared less and were more likely to shun Covid prevention after learning about the disproportionate ways it impacted (and is still impacting) Black communities and other communities of color.[13]

This happened nearly everywhere—not just the US. Covid-19 continued to spread and reinfect, evolving and mutating, reinfecting without limits and getting better at everything it does. The primary reason fewer people immediately die from Covid now than in 2020 is from vaccination, not "milder" variants.

A mountainous shadow of Covid's death toll looms over us and grows daily yet goes unacknowledged on every level. In May 2020, the number of people in the United States who died from Covid-19 passed 100,000 and was described by *The New York Times* as "An Incalculable Loss."[14] By May 2022, in official numbers widely acknowledged as an undercount, the US crossed the unimaginable number of one million dead. That time, *The New York Times* ran, "U.S. Surpasses 1 Million Known Covid Deaths."[15] That same year, *The Economist* estimated "The pandemic's true death toll" with "95% confidence interval" as low as 18.5 million, and potentially as high as 35.2 million—globally.[16] The United States has never acknowledged its undercounts or deaths where Covid caused new-onset conditions. Long Covid has never been a pandemic metric.

In 2023, individual nations ended prevention efforts altogether and declared "Covid is over." Except Covid-19 would like a word. No single nation can just decide to end it. We are in the 5th year of an ongoing global pandemic while a tsunami of studies show in the bluntest terms that Covid's initial acute infection is just the tip of the iceberg.

Covid-19 is called a "novel" coronavirus because it's brand-new to us. We are learning as we go along. Children born in 2020 will never know a world without Covid and Long Covid, and we don't know what two infections a year will do to them by age 10. We don't know why some people get Long Covid, although reinfections and lack of vaccination play a part, and we have no idea if people with Long Covid will ever get better. We don't know if Covid-19 will kill someone outside of Long Covid after ten years from the immune system, neurological, and vascular damage it leaves behind in almost everyone it infects.

We do know a lot more about Covid now, though.

Covid-19 is airborne.[17] When a contagious person exhales, the air they expel has virus in it that can infect people who inhale it. Covid can hang out in the air of an unventilated room for several hours—at least five, per a 2024 study on hospital-acquired infections.[18] Think of it like smoke hanging in the air when someone puffs on a cigarette. Infection can happen quickly. Studies show that in poorly (normally) ventilated rooms, an unmasked person can catch Covid in as little as 20 seconds to four minutes.[19] It's one of the most contagious viruses on Earth. It is only safe for scientists working with SARS-COV-2 to do so under stringent precautions in a Level 3 biosecurity lab (BSL-3).[20] Other pathogens worked with at BSL-3 levels include H5N1 (bird flu), yellow fever, West Nile virus, and the bacteria that causes tuberculosis (TB).

You can't tell if someone is sick just by looking at them. Data estimates published in May 2021 show that 1/3 of people infected with Covid-19 show little or no symptoms.[21] They may not know they are infected, due to absence of symptoms and lack of testing. Hand washing only prevents the *least* common ways to contract the virus.

Vaccination and antivirals are your last lines of defense. We learned in 2022 that Covid boosters wane dramatically at around 100 days.[22] That's what happens when a virus is allowed to evolve and mutate. Vaccines help you fight the virus once you're sick, but do not prevent getting infected. There was a time when they might've, but Covid-19 was allowed to run rampant and it evolved, so that horse has left the barn. I would leave too, if I could. Take me with you, horsie.

Covid-19 shows up with flu-like symptoms but is not just a respiratory infection. Covid has two stages: acute (the initial infection) and post-acute. It is a multi-organ, systemic disease; researchers at Monash University in Australia concluded in 2022 that Covid is "a multi-system cluster bomb" with "considerable risks" beyond the initial infection.[23] "You are 15 times more likely to acquire myocarditis requiring hospitalizations following Covid-19 compared with beforehand," Monash reported, with highest risk "around 14 to 60 days" after an infection.

Post-infection heart problems are not rare. Johns Hopkins reported that "*anyone* infected with Covid is at higher risk for heart issues—including clots, inflammation, and arrhythmias—a risk that persists even in relatively healthy people long after the illness has passed."[24]

Covid brings the risk of brain injury. Per Harvard Health in 2023, "Unfortunately, Covid can damage the brain in many ways. When people first become sick from the virus, they may develop encephalitis—inflammation of the brain—causing confusion, difficulty concentrating, and memory problems."[25] They added: "Even if people escape brain damage during the initial attack of Covid-19, they remain at considerably greater risk of various brain conditions, including strokes, depression, anxiety, and psychosis for the next several years. People who were initially severely ill with Covid are at much greater risk for cognitive decline after they recover. Even people who were less severely ill remain at a somewhat greater risk. A large study of MRI scans taken before and then again after people got Covid showed that Covid can actually shrink the brain somewhat."

> "Well over 100 scientific articles describe immune system damage caused by Covid. This provides a direct causal scientific explanation of unprecedented outbreaks of many other diseases." —Yaneer Bar-Yam, co-Founder. World Health Network

Covid-19 causes harm to the immune system and increases susceptibility to other pathogens.[26] Getting infected does not "build immunity" to anything. John Wherry, director of the Penn Medicine Immune Health Institute, summed it up to *Kaiser Health News* in 2021, saying: "Covid is deranging the immune system in complex and deadly ways," adding that "the coronavirus unhinges the immune system more profoundly than previously realized."[27] Some researchers have labeled Covid "the autoimmune virus."

Despite what we were assured, kids are not "immune" nor does Covid go easy on small children. *New York Magazine* reported in 2021 that Covid's risk of severe disease, death, and hospitalization to children was "actually lower" than the flu.[28] There was no year-over-year data to back this claim.

By August 2024, Long Covid in kids was labeled "a public health crisis"[29] with *most* of them having orthostatic intolerance,[30] followed by a September 2024 report showing "children under 5 years old have a weaker immune response to Covid-19 compared with older children and adults."[31]

Pets get it, too.[32] By infecting your cat or dog with Covid-19, you risk imparting them with brain injury and delayed-onset, long-term harms.[33] Take my advice and don't read about the after-effects experienced by some cats and dogs unless you're mentally prepared.

> *"I don't think it's well understood that the number of people suffering from Long Covid is not just very large, but it's expanding. It doesn't have to continue." —Prof. Brendan Crabb (@CrabbBrendan, Aug 11, 2024)*

Long Covid can result from one or multiple reinfections, at any severity of initial infection. The CDC places risk at 1 in 5 people.[34] A Public Health Canada review found that "half" of Covid cases have it at 12 weeks.[35] The Mayo Clinic places incidence at 10-35%.[36] Typical onset time for Long Covid is 4 weeks after infection.[37] There is no treatment for Long Covid. There is no cure for Long Covid. There is no prevention for Long Covid. Anyone of any age or health status can get Long Covid. The rate in children is 1.4%.[38] 2024 estimates show that at least 400 million people worldwide have been affected by Long Covid.[39]

Every reinfection increases the risk of Long Covid.[40] The AMA wants people to know that getting reinfected is "akin to playing Russian roulette."[41] Physician Rambod Rouhbakhsh warned in an American Medical Association podcast: "Each subsequent Covid infection will increase your risk of developing chronic health issues like diabetes, kidney disease, organ failure and even mental health problems."

Speaking of health issues that increase risk... We've been told throughout the pandemic in the vaguest terms possible that only

THE COVID SAFETY HANDBOOK

high-risk people need to worry about Covid, like people who are immunocompromised. But what does that even mean?

Immunocompromised is when your immune system's defenses are low, diminishing its ability to fight off infections and diseases, like those undergoing cancer treatments, bone marrow transplants, people with type 1 diabetes, lupus, HIV/AIDS, rheumatoid arthritis, asthma, leukemia, lymphoma—oh, plus old age and smoking all count as "immunocompromised" according to Penn Medicine.[42] A growing number of people are now immunocompromised and have a weakened immune system due to Covid and Long Covid. Many immunocompromised people often have a lesser immune response to Covid-19 vaccination, or can't tolerate mRNA vaccines.

Multiple studies and surveys show that the burden of Covid-19 and Long Covid disproportionately affects Black, Indigenous, People of Color (BIPOC),[43] women, queer, transgender, gender-diverse,[44] disabled and chronically ill populations.[45] People with brown skin and women are the populations hardest hit by Long Covid. They are statistically found to be less likely to be diagnosed, due to medical gaslighting, racial discrimination, medical misogyny, and Long Covid gaslighting.[46] Reports, like the KFF Covid-19 Vaccine Monitor September 2023, show people of color are far more likely to take Covid precautions like wearing a mask, while white people are least likely among all groups to take any precautions at all.[47] This is critical in understanding how Covid-19 anti-prevention measures and barriers to Covid healthcare are centered on racial and class inequities—and straight-up racism.

Previous infection does not keep you safe. Omicron changed *everything*. Post-infection immunity shortened to 28 days, something researchers discovered in 2022.[46] This was reported in mainstream media outlets—but appears to have not become common knowledge.

WHAT WE WISH PEOPLE KNEW ABOUT COVID

In August 2024, the US CDC published its new Covid-19 Prevention Guidelines for Early Care and Education Programs. It recommended vaccination, disinfecting surfaces, staying home when sick, using "ventilation systems," and gave detailed instructions for hand-washing "frequently." There was no single mention of masks or masking, nor did the document inform ECE programs that Covid is airborne. Based on this, it's no wonder most Americans don't know how to avoid the next reinfection. This is just one of many examples of how public health leadership perpetuates (and acts on) inaccurate Covid-19 perceptions and information. Hand washing and vaccine-only strategies are for the flu. That's the wrong virus.

That guidance was issued during one of America's largest, longest-ever surges, with an estimated minimum of one million new infections every day, over the course of several months. While at the same time US health officials had yet to begin the release of updated Covid-19 booster shots. Simultaneously, the World Health Organization issued a bulletin stating that the rise in Covid cases is "unlikely to decline anytime soon."

> *"And we're still expected to take buses, return to office and go to cafes built like giant Tupperware, with zero mitigations, and hot-box each other's breath without a care in the world." —A*

Most people who've stopped Covid-19 prevention practices or do nothing to prevent getting infected are doing so because they've been misinformed or misled, they're exhausted or find it too confusing, and because we've all been abandoned into an information vacuum. Some people don't try to prevent their next infection because they've given in to hopelessness or helplessness. It's also possible that a few may have lingering or increased cognitive impairment from one or multiple Covid infections, affecting risk assessment and impulse control, or short-term memory loss. That impairment is real, and well-documented. This is all explored in the chapter "Covid Personality Changes."

For some, everything that's brought us to this point feels so personal, so awful, and so unfair. That's because it is. Having no safe spaces to go, risking death or disability for seeking healthcare, being gaslit by family and headlines, lied to by public health officials, and abandoned by leadership. On top of all that, we cope with getting rejected by our friends who've gone Covid-YOLO (as in, the popular acronym used as an excuse for ignoring negative consequences, "You Only Live Once"). It's painful. It feels like a violation of trust, our social contracts, and our boundaries.

What's absent is a baseline of understanding about Covid-19. Everyone believes something different. This part of the pandemic feels like someone combined the era when many people believed you could "catch AIDS on a toilet seat" with the time when doctors partnered with tobacco companies to tell the public that smoking was not only harmless, but actually good for you. What we need right now is just for everyone to know the basics about Covid.

Here's what we wish our friends, family, coworkers, and everyone knew about Covid-19:

• Covid is airborne; it spreads through the air (not just drops from coughs).

- Covid is preventable.
- Everyone is vulnerable regardless of age and health.
- It's in people's exhales; it can stay active in the air of an unventilated empty room for hours.
- Some Covid infections are asymptomatic, meaning the person doesn't feel or look sick.
- Vaccination does not prevent infection: it helps you fight one.
- Masking is your first line of defense.
- Vaccination is your last line of defense.
- You're contagious if your test is still positive.
- Contagiousness lasts an average of 7-10 days, sometimes longer.
- It is lethal for some people.
- You can get reinfected in as little as one month.
- Covid damages your immune system; heart or cognitive damage is not uncommon.
- There is no limit to how many times you can get Covid.
- Covid can trigger new-onset diabetes and dormant viruses.
- Long Covid can take 4-12 weeks to show up.
- Most cases of Long Covid come from "mild" infections.
- Anyone of any age can get Long Covid, even healthy people.
- We don't yet know why some people get Long Covid and others don't.
- Long Covid has no cure or effective treatments.
- Reinfection increases your chance of getting Long Covid.
- We don't know if everyone recovers from Long Covid.

You probably noticed that many items on the above list run counter to what many people know, or believe about Covid-19. As I'm writing this book, a September 2024 poll of US adults found that half of

Americans believe that after having a Covid infection they'll never get it again.[49]

Despite what we know about reinfections, millions of people are operating on old, outdated, or shockingly incorrect information about Covid basics.

Thanks to disastrous public health communication from leadership and shambolic, short-sighted pandemic responses around the world, myths about Covid-19 are pervasive and endure throughout all levels of society. Some of those widespread myths include:

- Covid is just like a cold.
- Endemic means it's over.
- Hand washing prevents Covid-19.
- Vaccination is all you need to prevent Covid.
- You don't need to mask if you're vaccinated.
- Only "high risk" people need to worry.
- Covid isn't airborne.
- Getting vaccinated once is enough.
- You won't get infected if you only lower your mask to eat.
- Masking doesn't work.
- If you feel fine you don't have Covid.
- People who are contagious look or sound sick.
- Covid has no lasting effects.
- A "mild" infection means you are fine afterward.
- It's seasonal.
- Kids don't get it that bad; kids don't get Long Covid.
- Covid is "mild" now; "mild" Covid is harmless.
- Vaccination makes you immune.
- If you have it once you don't get it again.
- An infection "builds immunity."

- Long Covid is psychological.
- "Healthy" people don't get Long Covid.
- Covid is "over" or "went away."

WE DESERVE BETTER

This book is an inclusive, all-gender, all-orientation, science-forward guide to physically, emotionally, and psychologically staying safe from our Covid-19 state of affairs, during a time when it seems like everyone thinks Covid is no big deal and are simultaneously sick all the time. Each chapter focuses on a different aspect of something that poses a risk, and functions as a navigation tool for the many very weird and upsetting situations we find ourselves in while trying to avoid catching Covid-19—or any situation that threatens to break us.

Some of these chapters feature explanations of prevention basics, while others contain sections ready-made for handing to a friend or loved one. This book warmly welcomes the friends and loved ones we hope to bring into the cause of preventing Covid-19, and also welcomes back anyone who stopped doing prevention and wants to pick it back up. There are many detailed guides to Covid and communication to be found here, with plentiful examples of what to say in different situations. You'll learn how to fend off gaslighting, safely keep your boundaries intact, and navigate tricky situations like travel and feelings of isolation.

This chapter ("Why We Stay Safe") is a basic snapshot of how we got here, with vital emphasis on disallowing revisionist history, honest discussion of Covid-19's risks and harms, and the obstacles posed to pandemic response by ableism, and racial and social inequities. In the next chapter, "Trust The Tools," we dive into prevention 101 and also set the stage for warmly welcoming everyone to join us in becoming prevention geeks. This chapter breaks down masks, air quality, CO2, vaccines, testing, and wastewater watching into easy-to-understand bites, demystifying jargon and making the tools less intimidating. A harm reduction approach to Covid-19 is explained so that all levels can be encouraged, and a section of advanced goodies and gadgets offers prevention extras more seasoned prevention practitioners may not be aware of.

"Plan It, Janet" is the chapter that follows our primer on prevention tools. This chapter is all about taking those tools and combining them to suit a wide range of situations and personal prevention styles. It begins with a focus on fostering situational awareness about Covid-19 safety and the elements of high-risk situations. Readers are offered a long list of example personal prevention rules for easier decision making, and a detailed walkthrough of how to do recon — to "know before you go" — so everyone's prepared for risks. Examples include indoor and outdoor spaces, travel (including planes and Ubers), and making hotel rooms safer. A clear, detailed example of what's in a Covid emergency kit and guides for isolation and recovery conclude the chapter.

The next chapter is "Covid-19 Boundaries." Readers will get an overview of boundaries and what makes Covid boundaries different from other personal boundaries, with a list of example Covid boundaries people use every day. This is followed by oodles of example boundary statements readers can use, from non-confrontational and gently educational to some that may come in handy when a firmer approach is warranted. People who try to push or weaken Covid safety boundaries are described in detail with examples of who Covid boundary pushers are, and what they do to try to make us take risks — like using emotional blackmail—and what to do with these boundary pushers. Readers are walked through different things boundary pushers might say and provided with multiple responses.

In "Talking About Covid" we look at just how thorny it is to talk about Covid-19 and delve into how to talk to friends and loved ones about it. This chapter is excellent for readers who want to bring it up or encourage someone they care about to be more careful but don't know where to start, how to guide the conversation, or what to do if it goes off the rails. You'll get some great goal-setting for conversations, ideas for non-confrontationally bringing it up and lots of sample conversation starters. Further, the chapter explores communicating with event organizers, services like healthcare, and people who invite you out. A look at difficult outcomes tackles when the conversation goes awry, like into misinformation territory, and keeping perspective when things didn't go how you planned.

The following chapter, "Covid Gaslighting," is a deep dive into understanding what gaslighting is, and the specific ways Covid gaslighting is weaponized to make us doubt the facts of the disease, Covid prevention practices and avoiding infection, and the exact ways Covid gaslighting occurs. Examples include being told we're overreacting (manipulation of reality), minimizing ("just the flu"), scapegoating ("pandemic of the unvaccinated"), disinformation and lying, and bullying tactics like coercion. Readers learn how to identify, assess, and act, with examples of situational Covid gaslighting. A complete rundown of societal and political Covid-19 gaslighting is explained, and a look at why Covid gaslighting in entertainment, TV and film is both personally hurtful and damaging to society.

In "Long Covid And Relationships" readers begin with an overview of what people with Long Covid can be experiencing in addition to physical symptoms: denial and disbelief, a sense of helplessness and loss, and the frustration and uncertainty that can affect friendships and relationships–along with an understanding of what partners may feel when suddenly thrust into the role of carer. An up-front exploration of what we wish everyone knew about Long Covid is covered in detail, followed by a look at one of Long Covid's biggest enablers, Covid-19 medical gaslighting—and how BIPOC women, gender-diverse, and disabled people bear the brunt. Next, an examination of Covid's cognitive and emotional symptoms, how these might affect relationships, and how to navigate avoiding stressors, as well as finding support outside the relationship that won't gaslight anyone. This chapter closes with what we know (so far) about what's being done to understand intimate partner abuse and Long Covid.

If you've ever wondered why a Covid-averse friend seems like they decided to stop being safe after getting Covid-19, then the chapter "Covid Personality Changes" is exactly what you're looking for. This is a look at how some people appear to behave differently after having Covid, and why that might be. We examine the concept of Covid and giving up ("eventuality"), optimism bias and exceptionalism ("I won't get Long Covid because I'm healthy), how risk-reduction outcomes like "I got it and I'm fine" morph into anti-vax beliefs, and when people retreat to binary thinking ("I can't mask forever"). This chapter also examines the virus itself as a potential cause for changed behaviors, examining post-Covid cognitive changes and how cognitive and mood-altering aftereffects of infection can influence impulse control.

"Isolation And Connection" is the chapter that addresses all of the factors conspiring to make us feel isolated and alone right now, all the really cool reasons we're actually not, and what we can do about feeling so damn outsider-y in our masks. Here we look at the situation of needing to stay connected while avoiding a disease that spreads socially, and balancing questions of risk-taking with what we need to do for our own mental wellness. We look at disability and social isolation, the "othering" of Covid-19 prevention, and—surprise!—the new togetherness of Covid prevention. Over 140 mask blocs around the world (and growing) means we're *far* from alone.

All of this affects us deeply. In "Make Anger Useful," we acknowledge how much we're struggling right now, and while bubble baths are nice, telling us to "practice self-care" by doing yoga isn't going to cut it. This chapter goes through the ways we're being affected internally by the ongoing pandemic and how that might play out negatively in our day-to-day so it can be recognized and addressed. We take a look at what to do when our feelings won't give us a break and how to find someone neutral and Covid-conscious to help with the emotional heavy lifting. Then we dig into why Covid-19 makes us angry, and how the systemic pathologization of anger forced on disabled people directly informs our experiences. Further, this chapter explores the different types of Covid-19 grief we're struggling to process and the meaning of disenfranchised grief in the context of Covid. Readers learn how to manage bad news and information overwhelm, ways to turn anger into (Covid-safe) action, and how to make a meaningful difference in turning this pandemic around by becoming a disability advocate.

Lastly, if someone wants to see your receipts, hand them the "References and Resources" chapter. This contains every reference, study, article, book, guide, resource, and tool described in each chapter.

This book isn't about "going back" to 2019 or "back to normal." It's about having the future we deserve.

TRUST THE TOOLS

> *"Masks, air filtration, and ventilation work against all variants. When we combine them with vaccines, treatments and adequate testing, we have layers of defense that work effectively together, no matter how the virus evolves. The key is to do it all, not rely on only one."*
> —Dr. Lucky Tran, (@luckytran, July 8, 2022)

COVID IS A SOCIALLY transmitted virus. It's in the expelled breath of infected people so sometimes it can stay in a room longer than people do. It mostly spreads when we do things with other people. To prevent getting it or infecting innocent people, we have to socialize, go to events, get healthcare, meet new people, and attend work or school differently than we did before 2020. For now, anyway. Covid-19 is preventable and its spread can be controlled, but that's not where we're at—not yet.

Prevention has been made way more confusing than it needs to be. If all you want to do is "whatever's easiest" I get it. If that's you, read the sections in this chapter about high-risk settings and masks, and then skip to anything else that looks interesting. With the basics of transmission and stopping the spread in hand, each of us can take staying safe at our own speed.

From the outside, air and mask quality info might look like rocket science to most. You don't need to know advanced air quality calculus, seek occult information on gadgets and air filters, or need to figure out what a "fit test" is to mask effectively. Countless individuals and organizations around the world have done all the hard work of nailing down how to stay safe from Covid-19 for us, in the glaring absence of accurate, accessible information from public health leadership.

If you're new to Covid prevention or are hopping back into it after a lull, you are warmly welcome here. You won't find this book shaming you for any reason, or telling you're doing something "wrong" because your prevention game isn't perfect.

This chapter is where you'll get the facts you need to prevent Covid, an easy-to-understand explanation of tools and how to use them, and a harm reduction approach to guide you through making the right decisions for your situation to help you protect yourself, your loved ones, and your community from Covid infections.

COVID HARM REDUCTION

Covid harm reduction is having the facts and tools to make the best decisions you can to reduce harm to you and those around you. Covid harm reduction starts with tough talk about the facts—knowing the harms and stakes of risk-taking—which is what we did in the first chapter. The next component of Covid harm reduction is a look at the tools that work best for protection. These come with clear instructions on how to do *as much as you are able* to prevent infection and spread. The final component is being able to tell high risk situations and decisions from those that are lower risk. That's risk assessment: a method for evaluating and navigating decisions in ways that prioritize reducing (or eliminating) risk.

The best way to reduce Covid-19 risk is through a layered approach: there are no magic buttons or silver bullets here. A universal Covid vaccine (aka "pan-coronavirus vaccine") effective against all coronavirus strains is still theoretical, though a few in development show promise. Until then, it's all about layering up.

Vaccination is only one of our prevention and protection layers. The "Swiss Cheese Model" of Covid-19 prevention is where protection layers are imagined as slices of Swiss cheese.[1] If Covid sneaks through one hole in one slice, it's most likely going to get stopped by the next slice, or layer, of cheese. The subhead for The Swiss Cheese Model of pandemic defense is "recognizing that no single intervention is perfect at preventing spread," taking into account that there is no one-pill solution (yet), that people aren't perfect, and that approaches like a vaccine-only strategy for a rapidly evolving airborne disease isn't going to work. A layered approach also acknowledges that Covid-19 prevention is a situational and class problem: peer pressure or anti-mask bosses, for instance.

Some people can try to be as perfectly Covid safe as possible all the time; they might have the privilege of being able to afford expensive prevention tools, work from home, and have access to the latest Covid information. Others don't have access to tests and face mask bans in workplaces; some might be struggling in high-risk relationships or have elements out of their control, like roommates or settings that invite mask abuse. Some readers may be struggling after five years of prevention best practices, trying to figure out how to make safe calculated personal risks while also balancing mental health needs and costs.

Until we get clean air everywhere and Covid-19 under control, risk elimination in daily life is reserved for the wealthy, privileged, or lucky. What matters is that you do what you can to reduce the chances of getting or giving Covid *when* and *how* you are able to reduce the risk, and never forget that it is your responsibility to not put others at risk.

But basically, the best way to protect yourself from Covid-19 is to assume that everyone else is infected and contagious until proven otherwise.

HOW TO: MASKS

Some kids like to play a game, possibly for the express purpose of rapidly aging their parents, called "The Floor Is Lava." This is when children climb on the furniture and pretend that the floor is a roiling sea of hot molten magma, and the only safe way to traverse the house is by avoiding contact with the floor entirely. Cats love this game, too.

I mention "The Floor Is Lava" because some readers may find it helpful for masking to imagine exhaled air from strangers, and especially air in all indoor spaces as "hot lava" but instead of magma it's neurotropic vasculitis with a minimum 10% chance of making you bed-bound potentially for life.

> *"I wish I could go back in time and know what a N95 mask was in 2021 and protect myself. I want to cry. I hate what my life has become. I am stuck in my house like a prisoner while everyone can live normally and*

enjoy their lives while I have to crawl to the bathroom on all fours." —Syd (@fcknsyd, Jul 2, 2024)

Masking has changed: it's time to get caught up. If you wore a mask for a while in the beginning of this mess and hated it, the range of comfortable masks available now (like disposable N95 respirators, which offer better protection than the chaos we had on our faces in 2020) will blow your mind. It may take some trial and error, but you will eventually find a mask that fits and matches your comfort level for safety—and your personal style, if you prefer.

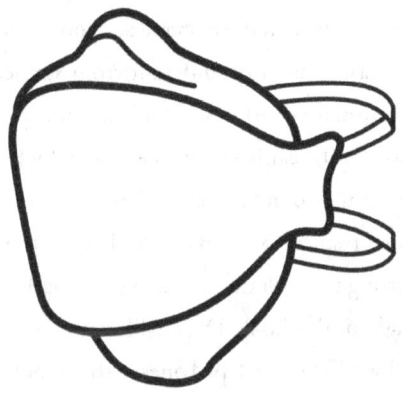

N95 respirator mask with two head straps

Here's a quick and important note on wearing masks for Covid-19: what you want is called a *respirator mask*. Per the 3M website, "Respirators–when worn properly–are designed to help protect you while you breathe in."[2] Surgical masks and other face coverings, they note, are for protecting others from your coughs and sneezes, though not from exhaled virus. So those disposable N95s (respirator masks) you see people in are preventing the wearer from catching Covid *and* from spreading it to others.[3] "Without exaggeration," *Scientific American* reported in 2023, "millions of people trust their lives to the effective 'real-world' science of respirators, with no need for randomized trial evidence."[4]

Surgical masks, like the green ones we see on hospital TV shows with two little ear loops, are what you're most likely to get handed when at the hospital. They're also what most people think of when they hear "Covid mask." We saw and wore a lot of surgical masks when Covid first arrived, before people knew more about airborne transmission and how incredibly easy it is to catch Covid. Unfortunately, those surgical masks you see some people wearing are leaking virus out *and* pulling virus in through the material and loose sides.

"Respirator masks" are a bit different from surgical masks. But when we say "respirator masks" we don't mean big plastic strappy spray paint masks with canisters on the side, which is what many people think when they hear "respirator." Some prevention fans have nicknamed N95s "respies" as in, "me w/my besties in respies."

We'll be referring to respirator masks as just "masks" (or "respies") for short throughout this book. Disposable masks are the most common ones you'll see, like cup-shaped ones with ear loops. Each person finds their own fit, durability, wearability, and comfort among all the options. Styles are generally categorized as "duckbill," cup-style, and flat-fold among the more-protective (respirator) range.

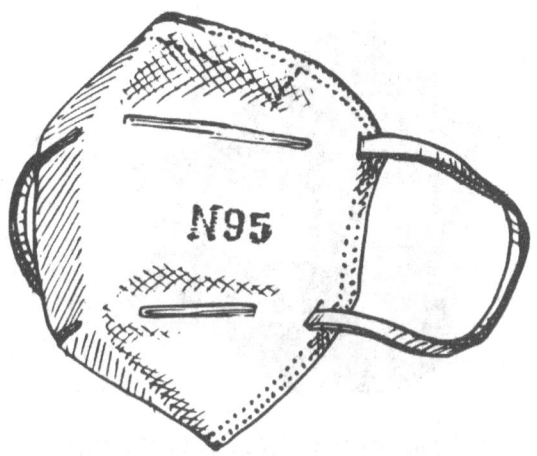

KN95 cup-style mask with two earloops

Some disposable masks have two straps that go around your head, others have two earloops. Some people really like the seal they get from head strap masks, and wearers tend to have preferences between smooth and braided straps when it comes to having short, long, or no hair. Head strap masks tend to come in higher protection ranges like N95 or N99; earloop masks come in a lower respirator range (KF94).

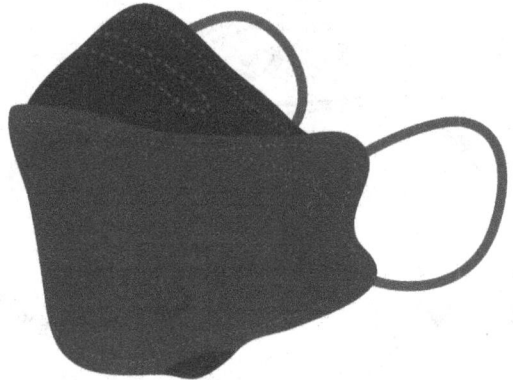

Flat-fold earloop mask in KF94/FFP2 style

Earloop masks are quick and easy to put on and take off, making them good for when you're changing environments. Some people always have one of each on hand, like using a head strap mask for the supermarket then switching to an earloop respie for walking home through the park.

Elastomeric masks are non-disposable, around-the-head masks; those worn for Covid-19 prevention are typically half-masks (covering the nose and mouth). They have replaceable filters, and in the case of the hugely popular Flo Mask, have filters for high-risk or low-risk settings.[5] The Flo Mask was designed specifically for Covid-19 prevention and has been worn by inventor Kevin Ngo and his kids for years, keeping them Covid-free even while traveling. An exciting subculture for Flo Mask decoration, cosplay, and fashion has emerged as well, like Mask Squad Cartel.[6] There are also snap-on 3D printed covers by steadirob.[7]

For detailed tests and reviews on more types of Covid-safe masks than can be listed here, look online for Mask Nerd, aka Aaron Collins.[8]

He makes yearly fit test spreadsheets and wonderful YouTube videos to help everyone—including kids—find "their" mask. Fit Test the Planet will give you detailed data on how your mask stacks up.[9] So will the Mask Together America Mask Chart.[10] Check the "References and Resources" chapter for these and more mask resources.

Masks need two things to be able to protect you: high filtration and a good seal. The 3M Aura is probably the most popular mask for Covid protection. That's because it combines high filtration with a great seal, and many wearers find them more comfortable than other options. But it doesn't fit every face shape (so doesn't completely seal for everyone), and some people can't tolerate masks with head straps. So if you can get a great seal from a KN95, which technically has a lower filtration efficiency, and also comes in ear loop versions, that mask will be the safer option for you because all the air you breathe will be going through the filter. If ear loops make it more comfortable to endure (or mean that someone is more likely to wear it in the first place), then it's also a fine choice.

> **Best protection**: N95 or better including N99, N100, and elastomeric respirators, like Flo Masks and Dentec
> **Good protection**: KN95, KN94, KF942, FFP2
> **Better than nothing**: Surgical masks, cloth
> **Worst**: no mask, a mask with an air valve.

That said, "proper masking" usually means wearing an N95 mask that fits so it's sealed on your face. This means no air leaks. But what if your work won't let you wear anything safer than a surgical mask, or a surgical is all you're provided?

Consider getting (or improvising) a *mask brace*, also called a *mask fitter* or *mask basket*. A mask brace fits over the top of a surgical mask to create a complete seal, similar to an outer gasket.[11] When your mask brace fits correctly, your mask will expand and contract when you breathe, and you won't feel air escaping around the edges.

If you need to get an MRI scan, you can probably count on healthcare workers to *not* be masking *and* to ask you to wear a flimsy surgical mask with the metal nose bit removed. This can be solved in one of three ways. One is to bring a silicone mask gasket to place over the surgical mask. A better solution would be to come prepared in a RediMask, the self-sealing N95 (no metal or straps). A third option is to use a Flo mask but change its head strap to a non-metal strap, like buttonhole elastic, which is a long strip of elastic with buttonholes sewn in, so it's adjustable.

Your mask doesn't get lifted or removed for conversation, making your coffee order at Starbucks, eating food, telling secrets, taking drinks, or selfies. (Although some people use an inhale-lift-selfie-re-mask-exhale technique, also used for security checks at the airport.)

Always mask indoors, in crowds, in stadiums, event centers, Ubers, the gym, at school, healthcare settings, at Costco, at Taylor Swift concerts, conventions, elevators, movie theaters, and especially around Olympic athletes and American politicians. The mask isn't worn on your chin or below the nose, because that would be silly. You would inhale hot lava.

HOW TO: AIR QUALITY

Air quality monitor numbers, types of HEPA air purifier filters, and calculating room size air changes is usually where most people's eyes glaze over and they decide that prevention is hard and confusing. If this is you, we are on the same team. Team AQ-WTF. Don't give up: a lot of very deeply nerdy prevention superheroes have done mountains of heavy lifting to make navigating Covid-y air spaces more like "choose your own adventure" than "pick your poison."

> "Pretty much all of the 'personal protection' approach described above is a stop-gap solution, until clean indoor air standards are developed and implemented. We are going through the equivalent of a 'boiling our own water' period for indoor air." —Prof. Brendan Crabb (@CrabbBrendan, Apr 26, 2024)

To be safe, we should generally assume all indoor air that isn't under our control has Covid-19 in it. It's other people's air: You don't know where that's been! Air with Covid in it needs to be changed by being removed (ventilation) or cleaned (air purifiers), ideally both.[12] Cross-ventilation is best because it removes all viruses suspended in the air. Ventilation can be opening windows and doors or running extractor fans, and air purifiers will continually change the air in a given space.

Look out for leaks in your clean air strategy. If you have housemates and can only keep the air in your room clean, make sure cracks around the doors are sealed when you blast your purifier and ventilate: this is especially important if someone in your household is infected.

The recommended rate to ventilate Covid-19 from an indoor space is 4-6 air changes per hour, but crowded rooms may need more (6 air changes means that the air is changed every 10 minutes).[13] If you have an HVAC system, use MERV-13 air filters.

Many people rely on air purifiers for Covid prevention. People have their favorite brands, like Medify or Coway, but what matters is that you find one that uses real HEPA filters and works for your needs, like being small and quiet or big, powerful, and pretty. The "ACH rating" tells you how many times the air purifier changes (cleans) the air in a given room. The accuracy of the air change rating depends on the room's size, so try to get a purifier that suits the size of the room.

Lots of people DIY their own air purifiers. An entire global culture has sprung up around making Corsi-Rosenthal Boxes (aka CR Boxes), decorating them for holidays and classrooms, and groups that host CR Box workshops for schools and community distribution.[14] These are efficient, effective, quiet, cost effective box fans consisting of 4 or 5 MERV filters, a box fan, and some tape.[15] What essentially started as Richard Corsi and Jim Rosenthal's Covid-19 safe-air social media tutorial grew into a movement, and now the Corsi Rosenthal Foundation provides grants and box-building materials, especially to underserved communities.[16]

Portable mini air purifiers make excellent companions—and they work.[17] The Medify MA-10, PureZone Mini, and others with HEPA filters have been shown in studies to help eliminate Covid from s paces.[18] It's important to remember that they're used to augment prevention strategies (not to be solely relied on).

Beware of wearable portable air purifier necklaces, which are marketed for travel. Wearable purifiers use ionization to filter pollutants out of the air, different to the HEPA filters found in purifiers effective against Covid. A study by scientists in China and California tested 4 wearable personal air purifiers, finding that 3 of the 4 removed less than 10% of particles in the air, making them ineffective against Covid-19. You're far safer in a respie.[19]

Far-UVC light is a technology that can virtually eliminate airborne viruses in a room, but it isn't a simple solution.[20] It's expensive, not widely available, and there are barriers to safe widespread adaptation, like the fact that you need to limit eye and skin exposure.[21] There are a lot of scammers and fakes selling lights that don't work to prevent viruses, or will seriously harm you. At this time, only one inventor in the world makes and sells a safe, tested portable Far-UVC kit and lamps for rooms: Nukit 222, also known as The Cyber Night Market.[22] Far-UVC is different than conventional germicidal UVC light, which can only be used in empty rooms because it damages skin and eyes.

MEASURE, KNOW, ACT

When we have to spend time in unsafe spaces it helps to have a tool that can give us an idea about the level of Covid-19 risk we're in, air-wise: CO_2 monitors. CO_2 levels matter because high CO_2 levels make the virus live longer and increase its transmissibility. More CO_2 means more Covid in the air, and that Covid is robust.[23] We don't have an exact way to measure the amount of Covid in any given space, but a CO_2 monitor can help us decide if a space is lower risk and safer to be in for longer periods, if it's a high risk setting and we should leave ASAP, or if a room is becoming increasingly unsafe over time.

CO_2 monitors come in different form factors (small and portable or large and affixed to a wall), and quality varies widely. Before going to an event or indoor public space, check online to see if the venue has any information about air quality; there are few, but it's possible to find venues that monitor CO_2 levels. Aside from that, consider adding a portable mini CO_2 monitor to your personal on-the-go prevention kit.

Mini CO2 monitors are essentially an indicator of how much "used air" is in the space, giving us an idea of how much Covid might be lingering and circulating. Popular models include the Aranet4, VitalightMini, SmartAir, INKBIRD, AIRVALENT, and the CO2.Click. All are battery-powered, fit in a pocket or bag, each has its own app, and all can be set to check the CO2 at regular intervals with results you can monitor on the app. Find reviews of mini CO2 monitors in the "References and Resources" chapter.

But what do the numbers mean in terms of Covid-19 in a room? Generally speaking, higher is bad and lower is safer—but when we say "lower risk" with CO2 we never mean "no risk." The low risk range will be when your CO2 monitor shows you numbers that match readings you get outdoors. Normal outdoor air is usually around 400. The lower Covid risk range for indoor readings is 500-800, though studies show risk is present in this range.

This range is ideal for masking up and staying for a show or a film, and it's what you want to see at the grocery store or other indoor settings. From 800-1800 is elevated risk; 1800-3000 and above is high risk. According to a 2024 *Nature Communications* study, "even with good ventilation, the probability of onward transmission approximately doubles for [CO2(g)] = 3000 ppm over the [CO2(g)] = 500 ppm after ~15 min of exposure."[24]

That's when you'll want to leave (or open all the windows) as soon as you can, or if you're trapped and can't go, this is when you'll be glad you're in a high-quality mask and prepped with any other prevention goodies or gadgets. It's common for airplanes to hit the high-risk range when boarding and upon landing, so don't forget to pack that mini air purifier in your carry-on.

HOW TO: VACCINES

Covid vaccines may not prevent us from getting infected, but they help fight the virus and lessen severity, and have been shown to help prevent Long Covid.[25] That's huge when we're at a moment when the only prevention for Long Covid is to not get infected, and we're pretty much only left with one treatment when sick: Paxlovid. Paxlovid is the brand name for a combination of two other drugs whose generic names are *nirmatrelvir* and *ritonavir*. Though we rarely ever hear it called by its generic names. It's usually just Paxlovid.

None of this situation is ideal. Covid-19 surges are year-round, each booster shot is calibrated for variants that peaked and left long before the calibrated shot was made available, and we learned in 2022 that Covid boosters wane dramatically at around 100 days.[26] That's just over three months of peak antibodies, followed by protection dropping off a cliff at 4 months. However, what remains will absolutely help you fight an infection. Until this situation rights itself, play vaccine Pokemon: collect them all if you can. Getting all the shots whenever you can *must* be part of your prevention strategy because every ounce counts. Always get a top-up.

HOW TO: TESTING

Testing is a powerful prevention tool. Taking a test prevents you from unknowingly infecting someone for whom Covid-19 could be fatal or disabling; testing can help prevent you from getting Long Covid if you catch an infection in time. It's always nerve-wracking. But testing is how we take action in being part of the solution—breaking the chain of transmission—rather than passively being part of perpetuating the pandemic.

You've probably heard a lot of things about whether or not tests work, or about tests and different strains of the virus. The at-home tests we all use now need to be updated, that's for sure. Those are called RATs (Rapid Antigen Tests) and when they're "positive" that's it, you have Covid. False positives are extremely rare. However, RATs are not great at being accurate about negatives, especially in the beginning of an infection or at the end. So you might take a test in the first few days after getting Covid and see negative results, which are false, or you might feel Covid symptoms and be totally perplexed by seeing the test say you don't have Covid.[27]

Don't worry: there's a solution. It's called *serial testing*. This is when you take a test roughly every 24 hours; serial testing in studies that overcame false negatives did three tests over 96 hours (four days).[28] It's no fun, but if you catch an infection in time for treatment and *don't* get Long Covid because you acted fast, or avoided accidentally infecting someone's kid... You'll be so glad you swabbed the decks (of your nose and/or throat) for a few days. Serial testing is the ideal but what's really important is that you do what you can.

RATs aren't the only kind of test you can take at home. Metrix, Cue, Lucira, PlusLife and other at-home molecular tests are expensive but much more accurate than RATs you get at the store. A couple of people I know discovered their positive status after following a negative RAT with an at-home molecular positive, trying the second test because their symptoms made them want to double-check. They deliver lab-quality results in about 20-30 minutes with accuracy up to 97%. Each has a portable electronic testing station (Metrix is the size of a small cell phone and charges via USB-C) and sells tests individually or in packs, and gives their results through an app. Test results can be sent straight to your doctor, GP, or telehealth consultant to speed up a Paxlovid prescription.

Like I said, molecular testing rigs and their tests are not cheap: at time of this writing, a Metrix reader is $50 USD and a single test is $25, while a Cue reader starts at $200 USD. This is out of reach for far too many people. You may decide it's worth the expense for much-needed Covid-safe time with friends and loved ones. I know a few people who keep a stash of these tests set aside for special occasions.

General tips: Always make sure to check the expiration date on any test box. When you test, keep in mind the following: blow your nose first, don't touch the swab on anything else, a swab with blood on it will be inaccurate, and if you eat, drink, chew gum, brush your teeth or smoke before a saliva test you'll need to wait 30 minutes.[29] Testing guidance has changed to include suggesting a swab of your throat (before you do your nose, ew) because it can give a more accurate result. Adding the correct number of drops is important for an accurate result.

Here's the final rule of test club: when you see a positive result, you're contagious—even if it's longer than the number of days you were told the infection would last. Most people are contagious for 5 to 10 days, but some will be contagious for longer.[30]

HOW TO: WASTEWATER

To get a pandemic under control and prevent as much death and disability as possible requires accurate surveillance and tracking, which has been a struggle and politicized mess with Covid-19 from the very beginning in most countries. At this point in time, few people know how to tell when the virus is surging. Publicly available data through official channels has oodles of data missing and plenty of bad policy decisions making numbers like cases and hospitalizations dangerously inaccurate.

For instance, on May 1 2024, the US CDC no longer required reporting of Covid-19 hospital data nationwide, yet unaware news outlets continue reporting that hospitalizations are low. By August, only 33% of US states submitted hospital data, down from 91% in May. Issues like this are not confined to the US. The result is that we have been abandoned to try and figure out for ourselves when it's safer to go out, or when transmission is high. Other than unreliable and infrequent headlines, it's practically all word of mouth and vibes at this point.

Almost. We can still look at Covid-19 wastewater trends and get a pretty good idea of how much virus is out there in our communities and cities, as well as observe trends, which helps us decide just how much to tighten our masks and rein in our risk-taking. Wastewater tracking measures how much Covid is coming out of humans and going into sewer water. It's only a general indicator, but measuring Covid danger in poop emojis is a pretty apt metaphor for where we're at. While measurement particulars can get confusing, websites that publish the data tend to put it into handy graphs so we can compare what it looks like now to what it was like when, say, Omicron first hit and the world has its deadliest surge to date.

Wastewater is another prevention layer for making risk-reduction decisions. Say you need to make a high-risk healthcare appointment but hope to do it when there isn't a massive surge going on. Check wastewater levels for your location (or as close to your location as you can get) and compare current levels with the previous six weeks, or six months. Maybe you need to travel and see family or go to a work convention in another city: time for a code brown! Check Covid-19 wastewater levels at the location you're traveling to so you can line up your prevention plan.

Websites in the US include Wastewater SCAN, Biobot, and the CDC; England isn't currently tracking wastewater but Scotland still does, Aotearoa New Zealand has the delightfully named "poops.nz" dashboard, and... you get the idea. You may not have Covid-19 wastewater tracking for your location or country, but it's worth a quick Google search to find out.

LEVELING UP

If you've spent any time in Covid prevention groups online or discussions about preventing Covid-19 anywhere, you've probably heard all kinds of bizarre things being tried or recommended. This is what happens when you abandon a population to a virus with no tools, support, or accurate information to prevent, fight, or even treat it: some people will drink horsie paste and chant. No one wants this! At the same time, scientific research on things like nasal sprays has quietly emerged showing results with different degrees of success in making Covid's life a little bit harder.

Below you'll find some prevention extras that have been tested and trialed, published data, and studies that specifically pertain to Covid-19 prevention—only. No supplements or herbal "cures." Anything in this section you decide to add to your prevention kit should be considered something *in addition to* masking, clean air, avoiding risky settings, vaccination, and testing. I am not a doctor and this is not medical advice. There is no substitute for the protection of an N95 mask.

Some of the things listed below are shown to improve recovery during a Covid-19 infection, and a number of people have added these to their prevention routines as a prophylactic measure.

Antihistamines are one example. Published in 2023 on NIH, a *Health Science Reports* article cited three studies, noting: "Several studies have shown that a number of Covid-19 patients improved significantly when on antihistamines due to their antiviral and anti-inflammatory properties. Moreover, antihistamines have shown to be effective in the management of long term symptoms post-Covid-19 infection."[31] Among those named were diphenhydramine (Benadryl) and cetirizine (many brand names, including Zyrtec).

You'll see lot of people in prevention circles recommending antiviral/antimicrobial nasal sprays.[32] A number of nasal sprays have been studied to prevent and/or treat Covid—some more than others.[33] Sprays containing nitric oxide or iota-carrageenan have been studied the most, in humans (not solely in lab conditions or just in animals), and with favorable results for treatment of Covid-19 infection to reduce viral load, and to aid in prevention.

Nitric oxide nasal spray, aka NONS, have been found to reduce viral load.[34] NONS have also been cited as a tool that "accelerates nasal virus clearance."[35] Popular brands include Enovid (an Israeli brand), FabiSpray, and VirX.

Nasal sprays, throat sprays, and lozenges containing iota-carrageenan "have been approved as common cold preventions and treatment and have been sold in more than 30 countries," according to massive 2023 analysis from international, peer-reviewed journal *Nutraceuticals*.[36] "A recent clinical study revealed that a nasal spray containing iota-carrageenan provided significant protection as a Covid-19 prophylaxis in health care workers caring for patients with Covid-19. Moreover, the German and the Austrian Society of Hospital Hygiene recommend the use of iota-carrageenan for the prevention of Covid-19." Popular brands include Agovirax, Betadine Cold Defense, Epothex, Flo Travel, Lontax Gola, and NoriZite.

Nasal sprays with ethyl lauroyl arginine hydrochloride (ELAH) sprays like Covixyl are often recommended and show promising results in animals in affording some protection.[37] Xylitol (brand name: Xlear) has been studied in people as a nasal disinfection practice against Covid-19 with good results, although it performed similarly to saline, differing in that no participants in one study using xylitol got Covid anosmia (loss of smell).[38]

Speaking of putting things in your nose... a 2024 study (on humans!) on Neosporin (neomycin) prompted some people to add it to their prevention arsenal when the study found intranasal application twice a day elicited responses that protect against Covid.[39]

The BLIS K12 oral probiotic has been shown in recent studies to produce oral and salivary antibodies that help clear the virus, similar to the salivary antibodies seen in someone after a Covid vaccination. One examined the use of K12 among infected people and did show a reduction of symptoms and surprisingly, in those hospitalized, "reduced the death rate in Covid-19 patients."[40] Another saw use in "frontline medical staff reduced the prevalence of respiratory tract infections by approximately 65%."[41]

Mouthwashes with CPC deserve further study. In 2021 the *Journal of Dental Research* concluded that "cetylpyridinium chloride (CPC)... reduces SARS-CoV-2 infectivity by inhibiting the viral fusion step with target cells after disrupting the integrity of the viral envelope. We also found that CPC-containing mouth rinses decreased more than a thousand times the infectivity of SARS-CoV-2 in vitro."[42] Further studies after the virus morphed into Omicron showed the same, also reducing the viral load in Covid-positive patients. One recent 2024 study in infected people found the opposite, showing no significant change in viral load.[43]

No one likes to end up talking to a "spitter"— and one of the lessons no one seems to have learned from the early part of the pandemic is to keep covering their sneezes and coughs. That's why a number of people add glasses or face shields to their layers. One fashionable, discreet option is a brand called Stoggles.[44]

While some mask decoration has been fit tested and shown to be safe, actually tampering with your mask is not recommended. Still, people with more advanced mask skills are trying the "Sip Mask."[45] SIP claims to be "an airtight valve that automatically seals after each sip." Installation needs to be precise, so please only try this if you can accurately test the seal for leaks afterward.

PLAN IT, JANET

> *"I went out last night to an event and there were a crazy number of unmasked people in a cramped art gallery, looking at me like I was crazy. The CO2 levels hit 1700 ppm. They were falsely reassured by the hand gel at the entrance. That's not how COVID spreads."* —Dr Satoshi Akima, (@ToshiAkima, Nov 27, 2021)

NOW IT'S TIME TO take the prevention basics from the previous chapter—masks, clean air, keeping an eye on surge trends—and all the optional gadgets and goodies, and map out your personal prevention style. This means getting your mask game together, making personal rules about situational awareness, and organizing your accessories. We're going to look at how all these things can be combined and used in real-life situations, as well as how to plan ahead for day-to-day prevention, events, and travel.

So much of surviving the ongoing Covid-19 pandemic has come down to anecdotes plus information and data sharing from trusted sources. In the vacuum of prevention from public health officials, we've had to step up to keep each other safe. We also need to stay sharp. I think we each have a story about recognizing a Covid trend as it emerges—like when breakthrough infections began occurring in vaccinated people after we'd been told that wasn't a thing—and then we saw data proving it. It became just another fact we needed to navigate around to stay safe, even if it wasn't yet front-page news.

No one planned for the pandemic to last for this long and none of us expected to have to figure out how to navigate a world that let the virus run rampant. But if those of us avoiding infection in a Covid-saturated world are anything, we're resilient. We adapt, we plan ahead, we stay flexible but have boundaries, and we're planning ahead. That includes everything from having an extra mask on hand in case one breaks to getting that booster shot (if they let us), as well as planning for things to go perfectly—and having a realistic plan in case they don't. We don't "move fast and break things." We've seen how that turns out. We move thoughtfully and suffer no fools.

If you're new to Covid prevention or are back after a break and realize some things have changed in how we avoid getting Covid-19, stocking up on better masks, air quality considerations, and prevention extras might feel a bit overwhelming at first. It's really a matter of just letting new habits set in. It won't be long until dashing on a mask before entering a supermarket is as reflexive as putting on your seatbelt before tapping the gas pedal.

Plan ahead and take time to familiarize yourself with your prevention gear and tools. Take a moment to check everything out, which is good to do anytime you get new masks or other prevention goodies.

Try on different masks and try talking, laughing, and smiling in them. Get used to taking them on and off, and find solutions for slippage or loose ear loops. One helpful suggestion for people who get panic attacks wearing masks in public or who feel claustrophobic in masks generally is to wear them while alone, starting with like a minute at a time, building up to 5 minutes, then 10 minutes, etc. It's a similar principle to getting used to wearing a CPAP (continuous positive airway pressure) mask for sleep apnea.

If you like the fit, colors, and feel of earlobe masks but the loops feel too loose to keep a tight seal, pick up some inexpensive silicone cord locks online, slip them on the loops with a paperclip, and cinch to get your just-right fit. Press the mask's metal nose bridge to shape it to your face so it's comfortable. This all becomes second-nature pretty quick.

Some people love their masks but worry about keeping the seal while going about their day wrangling kids or just dealing with humans generally. That's when garment tape—known for keeping Hollywood red carpet dresses from becoming wardrobe malfunctions—comes in handy. Another option for added comfort and seal are cheap adhesive foam strips sold online.

Do a basic fit test by cupping your hands over the front of the mask, then inhale and exhale. You shouldn't feel any air leaking around the sides of your mask where it meets your face.

Are you trying out some snazzy protective eyewear, too? Try those on with your mask, too. If you're going all EDC (everyday carry) check out your mini air purifier's different settings, poke at your CO_2 monitor and look through the app settings, and decide what goes in pockets, in your bag, and of course, on your face.

PERSONAL PREVENTION RULES

A big part of Covid prevention is making personal prevention rules. Rules will help you shape how you plan everything from going to work and seeing friends to travel and going to events. Covid rules center on minimizing risk by avoiding contact with Covid-y air, avoiding high-risk settings, keeping masks on, and making boundaries that keep you out of situations where you'll be pressured to risk catching Covid.

> *"Y'all masking? Day 13 of an international trip, 2 flights, 3 long train rides and I can't count how many subway/metro/tube rides. Here our simple rules. 1. Well fitting masks when indoors 2. Patio/Outdoor dining only(or takeaway) 3. Open window in hotel/apt. when there." —Aaron Collins, aka Mask Nerd (@masknerd, Jul 8, 2024)*

Some examples of personal rules might include:

- I wear a mask when entering any other door than my own.
- I mask indoors with no exceptions.
- Indoor space is something I share with people in N95/respirator masks.
- If people are nearby I wear a mask outdoors.
- No crowds, even if I am masked.
- No indoor dining.
- I stay masked in school, even in hallways.
- Indoor, no-mask spaces have time limits.
- I only unmask outdoors around people who have tested.
- If someone outside my household is negative after a few days of serial tests, I will unmask indoors.

- I only see doctors who properly mask.
- No one gets in my home without an N95 mask.
- I have a threshold for my air quality monitor (like 1200) and leave when it hits the limit.
- When air quality is bad I step outside to put on a beefier respirator.
- I never lift my mask on airplanes.
- Outdoor dining is okay if away from crowds and/or supported by mask wearing.
- My friends and I test before and after hanging out.
- Flo Masks in the club, no substitutions.
- I only go to outdoor events.
- Everyone has Covid until proven otherwise.
- Indoor events must have high air quality standards.
- I wear a mask for walks with friends.
- Exposed household members must isolate until they test clear.
- A portable mini air purifier goes everywhere with me.
- I leave when someone tells me to lift my mask.

> "How do I use a CO_2 monitor in my daily life for infection risk? Some examples: Measuring the impact of steps like opening windows. As a prompt to turn air filters on or up. As a prompt to use another mitigation like UV-C. To know if I should leave. What do I not use a CO_2 monitor for? Deciding whether or not to take off my mask inside. To just watch it go up and up and not act to either reduce the potential aerosols in the air or leave. The reason I don't use it for these things is because I don't want to get sick." — Amanda Hu (@amandalhu, Apr 27, 2024)

THE ELEMENTS OF HIGH-RISK COVID SETTINGS

Let's get acquainted with what makes a setting high risk.

No one masking. It would be safer if everyone was masked because masks work in two directions, but you're greatly reducing your risk by masking when others aren't. A 2024 University of Maryland study (on people who were not instructed on how to wear a mask) concluded N95 masks "captured 98% of exhaled virus," with surgical masks, cloth and KN95s coming in at 70%.[1] Two people chatting maskless is a 90% risk of infection within a few minutes, per the Canadian Medical Association, who estimated someone in an N95 would be infected from chatting with an unmasked infectious person in about an hour.[2]

No ventilation, no air purifiers: Covid loves a stuffy room and "used" air. A 2024 study from the University of Bristol showed that Covid's lifespan and transmissibility is boosted by high CO_2 levels—it increases the chances that more people will be infected.[3]

Covid-19 lingers in the air after infected people have left the room. The longest it's been shown to hang in the air is 5 hours. According to a 2024 study published in *American Journal of Infection Control*, two patients admitted into an empty hospital room 2 and 5 hours after a Covid-positive patient left caught the virus, suggesting "that airborne SARS-CoV-2 may transmit infection for over 4 hours, even in a hospital setting."[4]

Outdoor proximity. Have you ever been around a smoker outside and accidentally got lungfuls of second-hand smoke? Yes: you can catch Covid outside. A 2023 study charted the course of an outdoor superspreader in a crowded night market, where "During their 1 hour and 4 minutes at the market, the index cases infected 131 people."[5]

KNOW BEFORE YOU GO

Take a chunk of stress out of Covid prevention by sizing up a situation before you're in it. Do as much recon as you can to know what you're getting into.

Take the Covid temperature of the location. The best way to not get Covid is to tailor your behaviors around the assumption that everyone around you is positive unless you know for a fact they are negative. You'll be around people who each have different ideas of Covid-19 risk and Covid safety. You don't know who is exhaling Covid. All it could take is one wrong breath. But with a little planning and a layered approach to risk you can make staying safe look (and feel) pretty damn easy.

Do your best to ascertain if there's a Covid surge going on, get as location-specific as you can, and suss out what you might expect on the ground. Is there a lot of virus circulating where you're going—or are Covid-19 wastewater levels amazingly low? If you're going into a Covid hotspot, then you'll know you should leave a room when your Aranet4 goes in the yellow zone, that empty rooms need to be ventilated before you unmask, and the hotel gym was probably where you caught Covid.

Say you're going to a convention in Los Angeles, California. Is the US experiencing a surge, or starting to? (Probably.) Officials always downplay even the worst surges while they're happening, so check discussions on social media and Reddit Covid-19 communities. Next, look at wastewater readings for California, and then specifically for Los Angeles.

Find out if the convention has any Covid safety protocols or protections in place, which may be under "Accessibility" on their website, or the venue's website. See if the venue's indoor spaces have information on ventilation of HVAC air filtration, and if there are any outdoor areas for socializing.

> "My C19-precautions are actually pretty simple (N95 indoors, in crowded, close-proximity conditions outdoors etc) but there is a caveat built in: if I am with someone takes MORE precautions than me, I automatically defer to them and do whatever makes them most comfortable." —LD

> "Ruthless masking. I've done two 4 day conferences. N95 at all times indoors including flight. I went outside to eat and drink, and made sure to have outdoor dinner reservations each night, which my coworkers were happy to accommodate." —LC

Finally, see what happened with Covid-19 at the convention last year: did hundreds of people get Covid at the con? Did the conference get a "Covid-Con" nickname? Do you think you might succumb to peer pressure and drink in a bar unmasked? Are you a smoker? Will your boss expect you to eat dinner with the team? At any convention, plan to test daily and pack extra tests accordingly.

Now assess the risk: if it looks like you're paying a visit to the red flag factory, prepare for heightened prevention and high risk, or make the hard decision to save the date for next year. Either way, be prepared to deal with a lot of people who don't take Covid-19 seriously.

Is it an indoor space?

A good indoor setting will have ventilation, like open windows or doors, or an optional outdoor area. A safer indoor setting will have ventilation or air purifiers, masks required, and a bonus would be tests required as well. The least safe settings are enclosed indoor spaces with no ventilation, no masks, lots of people or crowds, places where there are sick people like healthcare scenarios, and have activities like eating, drinking, dancing, yelling, or singing. You want to avoid these settings or spend the least amount of time in them possible.

> *"I keep a carbon dioxide monitor with me in meeting sessions. Normally I wear a loop mask (KN95) but switch to an N95 if CO2 levels are higher than about 700 ppm."* —J

Some indoor locations and entertainment venues might have HVAC with air filtration: you may be able to find out before you go. Will anyone be masking? If not, add this to the risk column and plan to wear a heavier-duty mask, like a 3M Aura. Think about how long you'd like to spend in it, and how little you can stay if it's a bad Covid scene. If you have to stay in an environment that's not ideal, consider bringing a portable air quality monitor so you can keep an eye on the CO2, and also consider bringing your own environmental tools, like tucking a mini portable air purifier in your bag.

Is it an outdoor space?

Find out if it will be possible for you to be distanced from clusters of people or crowds. Outdoor spaces are much safer than indoors but you can still catch Covid outside: don't forget that that study where one person infected over 100 people in an hour was done at an outdoor night market.

Will you be seated close to other people in an outdoor crowd, like at a baseball game? Mask that pretty face! Because if you had an outdoor brunch and sat next to someone who is positive, even if showing no symptoms, you have been exposed.

> *"KN95+ at all times in public spaces incl drive thrus; don't eat indoors or on patios; friends who hang out with me and don't mask I ask to test beforehand + send a pic (I still mask the whole time); when I remember, I use nasal spray before going into mandated indoor spaces; test 1x per week."* —L

How are you getting there and back?
Travel and transportation are situations we have less control over, but that doesn't mean we can't stay safe and be prepared to get stuck in an unsafe situation for periods of time. When taking an Uber or taxi, keep your mask on and crack at least one window—also consider packing your mini air purifier if it's a long drive or you might get stuck in epic traffic (like going six blocks in NYC). Same goes for buses, trains, and subways: don a burly mask for heavy duty and keep it on. Ideally, sharing a car with a friend or carpooling would be an occasion when you'd ask everyone to mask up, but all you can do is ask.

Traveling by plane is high risk. No one masks, people are traveling while sick, and CO_2 spikes during boarding and deplaning—periods in which you might get stuck sitting for an extended amount of time. In a 2024 review of airplane flights and Covid infections, flight duration correlated with Covid infection risk. Long flights (6 hours or more) significantly increased risk (25x): "long flights with enforced masking had no transmission reported."[6]

> "US-Sweden: 4 airport/plane: nose spray, nose filter, CPC mouthwash, N95 w sip mask (cover on); personal air purifier. 4 hotel: 200 sq foot air purifier, carried in luggage, covered hotel vents w Redi-masks, windows open, no indoor dining, no crowded out door spaces."
> —L

> "N95 mask in airport/plane. To eat, switch to KN95 and lift up briefly and put back down. As much outdoor dining as possible—if forced inside, same mask trick. Spend most time outside, put mask on for quick trips into stores/museums/whatever." —E

Research from 2018 on viral transmission on commercial airplanes found that window seats are the safest seats from germs on a plane because they're the most isolated.[7] A 2022 study on optimal seating to avoid Covid-19 concluded that "the most dangerous seats are the seats next to the infectious passenger and the rows behind the infectious passenger."[8]

For plane travel, wear your most protective mask and plan on declining food and drink service—although some people do the inhale-lift mask-sip-lower mask-exhale trick, which is edgeplay if you ask me. Buff up with any nasal sprays, lozenges, or other tricks up your sleeve before you enter the airport, and strongly consider keeping a mini portable purifier in your carry-on bag. Then keep it in your seat with you. You'll be made to lift your mask for security: try to inhale-lift-lower-exhale quickly. If there's a chance you might fall asleep on the plane, take steps to ensure your mask will stay on.

> "I wear a headloop FFP2 mask and don't drink or eat anything. If I am asked to show my face, I hold my breath." —B

Where are you staying?

Are you staying with friends or family, in an Airbnb, or a hotel room? Consider potential risks in each of these settings. Are your friends or loved ones on the same page about taking Covid-19 seriously—or not? Get advice, templates of what you can say, and pointers on how to find out and navigate prevention conversations in the "Talking About Covid" chapter.

A rental (like an Airbnb) will most likely be the setting you have the most control over. When you check in, air the place out completely and set up your little Covid safety station (masks, charger for your purifier, etc.). Scope out whether there are any areas around the rental where you might share air with neighbors, like a building hallway or entry.

Hotel rooms take more work and come with more risk—though having someone else wash your towels is pretty wonderful. Do your best to get a hotel room with windows that open—many do. Every time you enter the room you'll want to change the air completely, from first entry to evening return, because there will have been people in your room that were unmasked and Covid can live for five hours in an empty room. Check for shared vents and adjoining doors: seal those with tape or magnetic vent covers if you can.

During an emergency evacuation last year—which happened to coincide with a Covid-19 surge—I was forced to move myself and the cats into a string of hotel rooms and short emergency rentals. When in a new room, I'd completely ventilate the space and blast the air purifier for an hour. While I did this, I checked the new space for connected doors, which got sealed with tape, and placed magnetic covers over vents between rooms. In one instance, the people next door spent their TV time next to an open vent that came through into my room. And someone over there had a cough. The cats and I survived the entire emergency evacuation without a case of Covid.

Some Covid cautious people have been known to ship a small air purifier to their hotels ahead of their stay so they can keep one continually running in the room. Don't forget to keep your mask on in hotel hallways and elevators.

> "N95 Aura, CPC mouthwash, Xlear, sanitizer for hands, sanitizing wipes for seats & tray tables, pure enrichment air purifier." —S

> "We've only taken 5-6 hour trips, but wore well-fitted 3M Auras or Flo Masks. Never removed from before the airport to destination. well hydrated for a couple days before travel & day of trip & ate well before leaving. Brought Pure air purifier 4 flight. Wore prescription Stoggles in flight." —G

YOUR COVID EMERGENCY KIT

With a nonexistent Covid-19 response from leadership and healthcare systems, we've been tossed into the churn to fend for ourselves. It's a brutal time for all of us. We're on our own, scrabbling for accurate information, comparing notes, forming emergency care circles, and trying to educate as many people as we can. That's true for everything from Covid transmission and prevention to dealing with infection and post-infection, as well as Long Covid.

Make a contingency plan for testing positive. You'll want to have everything at hand so you don't have to navigate a fever, brain fog, or panic to get in touch with your doctor (if you have one), or figure out if you can get Paxlovid in time. If you're traveling, find out if your hotel has concierge medical services and how the hotel assists Covid-positive guests.

Read this Covid Emergency Kit guide as a list of suggestions. Try not to feel like you "didn't do enough" if you're not able to (or can't afford to) get everything on this list. Thanks to the "you do you" mentality—a pandemic-prolonging individualistic response to a collective problem—we've been made to feel as though we'll never be able to do enough to prevent infection. That getting infected is our fault. That being denied medications is our fault. That not being able to afford air purifiers and nasal sprays is our fault. Even asking people to mask up somehow makes it "our fault" that they had to remember Covid isn't "over." None of this is our fault.

> *"Some will say you're overboard for the precautions you've taken to date. Others will say you failed and must've done something wrong to get it. Ignore. You've made many sacrifices. Keep up the good work. Improve where you can, and do what you can to delay a*

2nd infection." —*Noha Aboelata, MD (@NohaAboelataMD, Jul 29, 2024)*

It's smart to prepare for illness; it's important to plan for Covid-19. If you live in an earthquake zone, you have an earthquake kit. If you live in a flood zone or a fire zone, you have an emergency evacuation kit. Since we've been forced to live in nonstop recurring mass reinfection cycles of a highly contagious deadly and disabling disease (every location is a Covid zone) here are some ideas for preparing your Covid Emergency Kit.

This guide is a starting point. Just as we use layers of protection, we use layers to fight the infection. You may already have some of these items on-hand; you may also notice some of these things are for Covid prevention—it all serves to fight back the virus.

EMERGENCY KIT

• Paxlovid: it works.[9]
• Metformin: a two-week course has been shown to reduce the incidence of Long Covid, reduce viral load, and potentially limit contagiousness.[10]
• Thermometer.
• Pulse oximeter: To help determine if a hospital visit is needed.[11] Pulse oximeters may overestimate by up to four points if you have Black or brown skin.[12]
• Air purifiers with HEPA filters: Reducing the amount of virus in the air aids in recovery and helps protect your household.
• CO_2 monitor: High CO_2 increases Covid's survival in the air; a monitor will tell you when to open a window or crank up the purifiers.

- Extra Covid tests: You'll need several on hand to avoid false negatives, for testing to exit isolation (a positive test means you are contagious), and to serial test after your first negative. Recommended serial testing is three tests over 96 hours. You may also be contagious for longer than expected.
- Masks, N95 or better: For you and everyone around you.
- Antihistamines: per NIH, "a number of Covid-19 patients improved significantly when on antihistamines due to their antiviral and anti-inflammatory properties. Moreover, antihistamines have shown to be effective in the management of long term symptoms post-Covid-19 infection."
- Antiviral/antimicrobial nasal spray; some nasal sprays have been shown to support Covid recovery, like nitric oxide nasal spray (Enovid, FabiSpray, VirX), ethyl lauroyl arginine hydrochloride (Covixyl), xylitol (Xlear), and Iota-carrageenan (Agovirax, Betadine Cold Defense, Epothex, Flo Travel, Lontax Gola, NoriZite).
- Lozenges: the BLIS K12 oral probiotic has been shown to produce antibodies that help clear the virus.
- Mouthwash: Mouthwashes with CPC can decrease Covid infectivity.
- Water and electrolytes.
- Cold medicines and over-the-counter symptom relief.
- Pain relievers/fever reducers.
- Ice packs.
- Low effort comfort items to pass the time: things to watch, podcasts, audiobooks, coloring books, games.

KNOW BEFORE

- Your doctor's contact information.
- Make a list of your medications and med schedule.
- Sick days and time off.
- Telehealth options.
- Social supports for help in isolation, getting groceries and prescriptions, and wellness checks.

KEEP IN MIND

- Average contagiousness is 5-10 days but can be longer.[13]
- Serious rest is recommended: that means rest from screen time, too.[14]
- Long Covid onset is typically 4 or more weeks after infection.
- Get boosted to help prevent Long Covid and help fight the infection.
- One test to exit isolation won't cut it.
- Serial test three times over the course of four days after your first negative result to be sure.
- Reinfection is possible in as few as 4 weeks.[15]

Make a physical isolation plan for your household. You will need to reduce virus in the air (purifiers, ventilation) throughout the house and block infected air from traveling. Try to place an air purifier in every room of your house, if possible. This can include sealing doors and vents, in addition to configuring and coordinating bathroom access to keep contaminated air from other rooms. Decide which rooms will be safe zones for uninfected people and which is the isolation zone (a bedroom). Coordinate a strategy for safe food delivery or access.

These guides can help you prepare:

- What to Do When I Have Covid (Clean Air Club)
- What to Do if You Have Covid (People's CDC guide)
- What to do if you get Covid (Monkeys on Typewriters)
- What To Do If You Catch Covid (Roots Community Health Center video series, YouTube)
- Someone in my home has Covid. How do we isolate safely? (Clean Air Crew)

COVID BOUNDARIES

"I love to see a Covid-conscious queen setting boundaries." —M

OUR COVID-19 BOUNDARIES ARE at the heart of staying safe and preventing infection. Yet we're years into an ongoing pandemic of a highly contagious virus, and due to lack of education and support for prevention, so everyone has wildly different approaches to Covid risk management. With prevention restrictions and social pressures, it makes sense that people's choices are varied. So it's important to learn about Covid boundaries, how we feel when we set them, what can threaten them, how we respond when we come up against other peoples Covid boundaries, and boundary pushers.

When a situation or a person puts you at risk for a Covid infection, it's not a joke. It's a serious health threat that can impact your body's ability to function normally for the rest of your life. That person or setting is a risk to your health and well-being. Yet some people will try to make you feel like you're asking too much by setting boundaries or like you should feel ashamed for asking someone to respect your limits. Others will tell you that getting infected over and over is just the cost of being "normal," as if virus prevention is somehow abnormal behavior. Some might say you shouldn't go out at all if you want to avoid Covid, as if going to the grocery store and coming back with Long Covid is what we should all be doing.

Telling us our prevention boundaries are invalid and that we should accept infection is manipulative, illogical, seriously backwards, and just plain wrong. We don't deserve to lose our cardiovascular health, cognitive abilities, bodily autonomy, senses of smell or hearing, physical activities we enjoy, sexual function, short-term memory, GI tract functioning, pain- and sickness-free lives (if that was even a baseline if you're already disabled), ability to play with our kids, or the lives of our elders just because we want to do what everyone else does every day.

> "If somebody wants to hang out with me, we are going to be masked. Otherwise we're not going to hang out. This goes for relatives as well as old friends." —D

> "We mask (N95) anytime we're indoors with people not of our immediate household unless the person we're visiting has isolated for 6 days and tested right before we get together." —P

Just as masks and clean, Covid-free air are on the first lines of defense, Covid boundaries are like sunlight to gaslighting vampires. Covid gaslighters try to get us to risk infection by messing with our heads and blurring our boundaries. When you familiarize yourself with Covid-19 boundaries and how to make them work for you, Covid gaslighting becomes easier to spot, defeat, and its negative effects will have less of a chance of getting on top of you when you're feeling down.

WHAT ARE COVID BOUNDARIES?

Let's talk about consent for a minute. Consent represents the conditions under which you say "yes." To give consent, you need to know exactly what you're saying "yes" to. If you know the risks that come with your "yes," you can make an informed decision and give your informed consent. Informed consent requires that your "yes" comes with the ability to refuse; it is having a clear understanding of what your "yes" means, and its potential consequences.

Boundaries are limits: they are your "no." Think of them like personal rules. The rules that stand in the way of you getting a potentially deadly and disabling disease. Covid gaslighting is an attempt to violate your boundaries—to get you to participate in breaking your own Covid safety rules.

EXAMPLE COVID BOUNDARIES

- Masking indoors.
- Masking indoors and outdoors when in crowds.
- Being unmasked outdoors around people who have tested.
- Agreeing to unmask indoors with someone outside your household

after 3-5 days of mutual serial tests.
- Only seeing doctors who mask.
- Setting a threshold for your air quality monitor and leaving when it hits the limit.
- Not lifting your mask on airplanes.
- Outdoor dining only complemented with masks.
- Testing before and after time with friends.
- Flo Masks in the club.
- Only attending outdoor events.
- Everyone has Covid until proven otherwise.
- Indoor events must have high air quality standards.
- All travel is masked.
- Only hanging out with masked people.
- Exposed household members isolate until they test clear.
- A portable mini air purifier goes everywhere with you.
- Walking out when someone tells you to lift your mask.

It's stressful when someone or a situation challenges your Covid boundaries. Not everyone will feel comfortable establishing or re-establishing their boundaries. It's perfectly okay if you decide to skip an event or lunch because you don't want to deal with potentially defending your limits or having to bring up Covid prevention stuff at all. Avoiding a risky scenario or deciding not to deal with boundary pushers is one of the ways you maintain your boundaries.

> *"Make hard rules and enforce your boundaries 'hey! I'm doing Covid safety these days, which means I can meet outdoors but I'll need you to (mask/test)'. if ppl disrespect your boundaries, they're not for you."* —Julia Doubleday (@julia_doubleday, Apr 27, 2023)

EXAMPLE BOUNDARY STATEMENTS

- "Masking indoors is one of my rules."
- "If you want to come in I need you to wear a mask."
- "Hey, do you mind masking up?"
- "Here, swap your surgical for an N95."
- "I can stay inside longer if we open a window."
- "I can't stay inside when CO2 levels are this high."
- "I'd love to see you! Can we meet outside?"
- "I'm not doing indoor spaces right now."
- "I don't do indoors without a mask on right now."
- "Hey just so you know, I'll be in a mask when we meet up."
- "Meeting up sounds great as long as you don't mind me being the one in a mask."
- "Yeah, I really don't unmask unless everyone tests."
- "I'd be delighted to. Is there a remote option?"
- "I'm taking this year off from in-person events but would love to attend remotely."
- "Can we meet on Zoom instead?"
- "Looking forward to seeing you. I'll text you a pic of my Covid test before I leave the house."
- "My bestie and I text each other our tests with the dates written on them for a few days before we go goblin-mode with wine and Netflix. Can we do the same?"
- "Hey there, just calling ahead to find out if you have any Covid protocols in place. Are y'all masking?"
- "We'd love to come to the wedding! We have to stay Covid safe though, will there be any outdoor areas for socializing?"
- That's a "no."

- Text a pic of your Covid-negative test before traveling to visit relatives as a way to say, "I'm still taking this seriously and care about your health."
- "That's not an option for me."
- "I'll see you some other time, then."
- "By 'mask' I mean N95 or better."

"I always fly w my N95 Aura and Pure filter, have my Aranet with me always, only eat outdoors, try to avoid crowded spaces as much as possible. I politely ask if we can eat outdoors for work-related dinners-if folks won't/it's not possible, I excuse myself." —CS

"I just tell people that I'm an 'outdoor person' now. When I do indoor stuff, I wear an N95 mask that has a good seal on my face." —AP

"I wear my masks all the time. If I need to talk or go to a networking event, I wear my N95 mask. If it's a crowded event, I wear my P100 mask. I don't expect people to follow or give space. I have to do what's best for myself." —T

BOUNDARY PUSHERS

Covid-19 boundary pushers will engage in direct or indirect attempts to get you to break your Covid safety rules. There are any number of motivations someone will try to violate your boundaries. It could be that being reminded of Covid makes them uncomfortable, they inaccurately believe Covid "is over" or "just a cold," or they've decided that prevention is pointless. There's also the fact that everyone is dealing with things we don't even know about. It can also be that the person messing with your boundaries is a creep who treats everyone poorly and you should avoid them whenever possible.

Some boundary pushers may have deeper issues which can make them hostile, aggressive, manipulative, malicious, or even deceitful. When you recognize that you're in a situation where you're being targeted by someone actively harmful like this, get out of their blast zone ASAP. The bottom line with whatever motivates a boundary pusher (or boundary breaker) is that their behavior comes from a place where they care more about how your safety protocols make *them* feel than your feelings or your safety. They have also prioritized their personal comfort over the safety of their family, community, and strangers. And they are not your problem to solve.

Unfortunately, we're surrounded by all kinds of Covid boundary pushers right now. Recognizing the situation is essential to keep your rules intact and avoid the temptation to question yourself. Covid safety boundary pushers are people who:

- Organize events that ignore Covid safety protocols.
- Force workers into indoor spaces with no Covid-safe ventilation or masking.
- Tell you to lower your mask to buy alcohol.
- Make rules that prohibit masks.
- Are healthcare workers that refuse to mask.
- Claim they can't hear/understand you with a mask on.

- Use emotional blackmail to compel you.
- Ignore your request to mask.
- Take a mask but don't put it on.
- Lower their mask to talk to people.
- Show up at your door unmasked.
- Insist you take a sip or a bite of food.
- Host indoor-only events with no outdoor component.
- Ignore your request to meet outside.
- Ignore your request to test before meeting up; ignore your request to exchange photos of tests with dates on them before meeting up.
- Complain to friends, family, or coworkers about your Covid safety boundaries.
- Claim they tested but don't have evidence, like a photo.
- Harass, threaten, abuse, gaslight, use racist or ableist microaggressions, or manipulate you to violate your safety rules.
- People who "forget" to test or bring a mask.
- Use peer pressure, like the fear of missing out (FOMO), disappointing a friend or family member, or insisting no one else is doing it.
- Encourage infection for any reason.

ADDRESSING CROSSED COVID BOUNDARIES

Sometimes all it takes is saying "no" or restating your request for them to wear a mask, meet up outdoors, or show you their Covid test before hanging out. You want to be there for loved ones and friends, and no one wants uncomfortable coworkers or to look like a problem to the boss, or a grocery clerk you'll be seeing regularly. You may end up declining brunches, limiting your time with certain people or family members, or having to be the one to organize gatherings and meet-ups.

There will be times when you need to address the problem head-on. For instance, you might have to repeat your requests for someone to mask or test, and set a hard limit that includes not hanging out with someone unless they do. You might show up to meet and have someone pressure you in public, like trying to get you to dine indoors, while others are watching. There might be times when you choose to leave groceries or a bottle of wine on a store counter because you've been asked to lower your mask; you might have to leave a business when a receptionist or security guard tells you that there's "no masking" inside.

Some boundary and safety decisions will be awful. You may have to make the hard decision to find a new job where your Covid risk is lower, walk out on a healthcare appointment, or find a new doctor or GP. You may need to confront a friend who won't wear a mask after you've asked them to. Sadly, some friends or family members may stop talking to you or including you because they don't like your Covid boundaries. You may discover they meet up without telling you. This is incredibly painful and it's normal to feel rejection and grief—on top of anguish knowing they are making themselves high risk for Covid infection.

Personally, I have lost friends and have had to decline career-making events (two high-profile conference keynotes, for example) because the risk was too extreme to navigate and both conferences would not offer a remote option when I asked. In one instance, my keynote replacement tweeted about getting Covid-19 at the event, which was a terrible validation of a decision I didn't want to make.

Some of us have had to deal with public harassment and acts of physical aggression for masking. This is an ongoing risk while public health officials continue to stigmatize Covid prevention, refuse to model prevention practices, and encourage the normalization of mass, repeat Covid infection. Those risks are encouraged by public officials endorsing or enforcing mask bans—and leadership that does nothing to prevent mask bans. Leadership matters. Seeing a US President refuse to mask while contagious with Covid-19, a US CDC Director who refers to masks as "the scarlet letter," and a White House Covid Coordinator calling people who mask "fringe" all emboldens individuals to harass and threaten those of us avoiding infection. The best thing you can do when someone attacks you for masking or carrying around a portable air purifier is get away from them.

Having to address boundary pushers or violators, whether with gentle redirects or facing them head-on is stressful. It also feels like labor—that's because it is, this is work someone else is making you do. But it's work that must be done because the alternative is Covid-19's "Russian roulette" with potential disability, increased disability, death, or a life-altering heart (or other) condition. You may have to take some very extended "time off" from a friend, family member, or even consider separation from a spouse who refuses (directly or indirectly) to stop putting you at risk.

Asserting your boundaries and having your rules or requests ignored can be exhausting. At the end of the day it's perfectly okay if you just decide to avoid situations, stop engaging with boundary breakers, or choose to walk away instead of restating a request. You never need to explain your boundaries to anyone, and it's not your job to educate people who drain your energy and put you at risk.

SAMPLE RESPONSES

I don't know about you, but I feel like I have all these witty or perfect responses to Covid boundary violators in my head, constantly thinking of new ones, but sometimes when the moment comes... Something else comes out. It helps to think about what to say beforehand, even if it doesn't come out perfectly in the moment. While writing this book, I found myself in a situation where I was buying a bottle of wine from the store near my apartment and the clerk called over to check my age told me to lower my mask. And there I was, confronted by a situation I knew was coming at some point, and I blurted out the first thing that came into my head, which wasn't anything I'd thought of before. I said, "I can't lower my mask." Then I waited to see what she would say or do.

I didn't even think about what I'd say if she had asked me "why not"—but I did realize at that moment I was just going to go buy wine elsewhere if she insisted. I thought about a friend I miss who has Long Covid, so I didn't really care what anyone thought of me if I walked out. I pulled out my ID card and she accepted it, so I found out that simply saying "I can't" works quite well. Most people are averse to confrontation, and I think this helped move the situation to a swift resolution.

They say: "Take off/lower your mask." You might say:
- "No." / "No, thank you." / "Nope, I'm good." / "Not today."
- "I think I'll keep it on."
- "Sorry, no can do."
- "I can't take off/lower my mask."
- "It's better for everyone if I keep it on."
- "Doctor's orders."
- "Sorry, personal rule."
- "Better safe than sorry."
- "But I look so good in a mask."

If they insist or ask why, suggestions include:

- "I'd rather not."
- "I can't afford the sick days."
- "None of your business."
- "Personal reasons."
- "I can't get Covid again."
- "I'm high risk."
- "I spend time around medically vulnerable people." (This is true for every public space.)
- "My [bestie, loved one] is high risk."
- "Everyone is sick right now."
- "Long Covid scares the crap out of me."
- "Why are you asking?"
- "This isn't worth getting Covid."
- "Covid levels are too high right now."
- "Because Covid is bad, actually"
- "I'm immunocompromised." (If you are comfortable disclosing.)

They say: "I don't need to [mask/test/meet outdoors] because [I feel fine/I'm vaccinated/I already had Covid]." You could say:
- "I'd prefer it if you do."
- "Then maybe we should do this another time."
- "I need to be really careful, so if you don't want to I have to make different plans."
- "That's too bad. Can we Zoom instead?"
- "I wish it was that simple for me, but it's not. I'd be happy to talk about why that is if you want to, but either way let's make a different plan."
- "No offense, but I think your info is out of date. I can't risk it, so

maybe another time."
- "Let me know if you change your mind."

They ignore your request to mask, test, ventilate. You can tell them:
- "Do you need a mask? Here, I have an extra."
- "Hey, are you going to put that mask on?"
- "So are you deciding not to mask?"
- "I seriously need you to wear a mask."
- "Can you put your mask back on?"
- "I forgot if I already asked: could you wear a mask for this?"
- "Don't forget your nose."
- "You know the nose sticking out is a meme, right?"
- "So if everyone doesn't test then someone might get me sick and I can't risk it."
- "Just FYI, I haven't seen your test so I'll be masking/staying outside."
- "Hey I didn't see if you sent a pic of your test, did I miss it?"
- "I'd love to be able to relax and spend time with you. The best way to do that is if you test for a few days before we meet up. I'll text you mine, just reply back with yours and we're all set."
- "Do you mind if I open the window?"
- "I'd feel better/be able to stay longer if we get some air through here."

Another common boundary-pusher tactic is "I can't hear you" or "I can't understand you at all with that thing on." Some people who say this will certainly be trolls, but others—like Deaf and Hard of Hearing (HOH) people—genuinely do have trouble hearing and understanding someone wearing a mask. One way to respond might be to say:

"I really can't, but I understand. Would it be better for you if I typed what I want to say and you could read it off my phone?"

Having Covid boundaries and a thorough knowledge of how to blend your protections and boundaries into life isn't just self-care: it's a refined, fun, mindful, and crafty way to move through the world and enjoy it safely. Never beat yourself up or feel ashamed because you're "the one in the mask" or decide to skip someone's wedding because it has all the hallmarks of a superspreader. It may feel sad to skip the family dinner this year because no one's taking Covid seriously at home, but maybe you can next year.

Don't forget that saying "no" now and avoiding Long Covid risk means you will still be physically able to attend a future dinner. Don't ever feel ashamed of saying "no thank you," boundaries and all. You are not fussy or demanding, you are simply someone with limits.

Never let people who don't understand make you feel bad or attempt to emotionally blackmail you into doing something unsafe. Never forget that you're not alone.

Don't feel lonely because you understand Covid-19 risk and transmission better than most people. You're way ahead of the rest of the world right now for keeping up with studies, wastewater readings, the latest findings, and for caring about the effects this disease is having on people. You are self-reliant with your own safety and make spaces safer for others—especially people who can't do it themselves. You know how to share your time, tips, tricks, advice, and personal space with other people when they take your boundaries seriously—and when they're deserving.

Relish your Covid boundaries. Your Covid limits are a gift. They filter out risks and jerks in equal measure. They keep you out of trouble—so someday you can get into good trouble, on your terms. Love your masks and limits, roll with it and even if you feel lonely make yourself feel good once in a while with a masked selfie or telling someone else their mask looks great.

Love your Covid boundaries.

TALKING ABOUT COVID

> *"Long covid is impacting so, so many of us in tech but it's like we're not allowed to talk about it. Major solidarity and appreciation to those who share, it makes me feel so much less alone."* —Dr. Cat Hicks

TALKING ABOUT COVID IS stressful. Even just thinking about talking about Covid is stressful. There are several reasons why in many settings the topic of Covid feels more taboo than porn, even in places where talking about disease prevention shouldn't be an issue. We never know how someone is going to react when we do have to talk about it, most especially when we're trying to assess risk, make prevention inquiries, or keep loved ones safe.

One reason the very subject of Covid feels like a parking lot full of landmines is that institutional leadership keeps hammering on the message that "Covid is over" while we damn well know it's not. Remember: no one is "just lucky" in avoiding Covid-19 or somehow immune to getting infected. The only way to avoid the cycle of Covid reinfection is to be consistent with your prevention protocols and boundaries.

Many of us don't like the way we're treated for being pro-prevention and risk-averse when the subject comes up. It's beyond infuriating to ask if a healthcare practitioner will wear a mask and hear them say they just "don't want to talk about it anymore." It's worse when a vulnerable family member tells you they're about to take a risk that will very likely get them infected, only to be rebuffed about any Covid prevention discussion whatsoever.

Covid is a stressful topic because it's risky. We never know if someone is going to be hostile, cruel, confrontational, or physically aggressive. There are other risks that hurt, too: rejection, loss of friendship, rifts in relationships, family members pushing us away or shutting us out, and sometimes we face hard choices. We risk having friends, lovers, and family members putting us in the position of choosing between their beliefs and our Covid boundaries.

Bringing it up, such as when disabled and high-risk people ask for healthcare accommodations like masks, brings the risk of being mistreated or "fired" by their doctors/nurses when the mask ask is perceived incorrectly as aggressive towards staff. This risk extends to our care relationships—parents, partner, or attendants—who might lie about precautions and spread illness to us, hurt us on purpose, or neglect us. It can also mean risking the loss of a doctor's appointment, rideshare, a child's playdate, or even a job.

Oftentimes, just by showing up in our masks we are *de facto* seen as the ones bringing it up whether we mean to or not. And we usually don't! We just want to get our groceries or get through our appointments masked and unhassled. Ultimately we can only guess at why someone won't engage with us about Covid—denial, misinformation, resignation, fear, grief, racism, ableism, discrimination, displaced blame and anger—but all of it remains as a direct challenge to our Covid safety boundaries.

No matter what, whether asking a doctor to mask or asking an event to move outdoors, you're going to have to be the one to bring it up. You might receive a mixed reply: part understanding, part hesitation. You may be met with a reluctance to talk about it, or you might receive an outright refusal. You may have to deal with teasing, ridicule, rudeness, someone Covidsplaining misinformation at you, hostility, or manipulation tactics designed to get you to violate your own boundaries.

Talking about prevention is easier if you're already someone who has other people in your life to talk to about Covid-19 prevention topics. It can be frightening if you never talk about Covid or if you're dealing with a situation where someone has power over you. This chapter is where you'll find out how to talk to loved ones about Covid, how to bring it up, advice for when your partner's risk threshold is different than yours, talking to kids, communication with events and businesses, and talking to people who want to be safer but don't know how.

HOW TO BRING IT UP: FRIENDS, FAMILY, AND LOVED ONES

Asking someone to be safer, take less risks, or warn someone about how dangerous Covid is will always feel charged and nerve-racking, thanks to all the creeps who've made Covid a divisive and misunderstood topic.

It might be that you're worried about a parent who believes some of the common Covid-19 myths. You may have friends who don't take precautions and you'd really like to hang out with them. It could be a roommate that keeps putting the household at risk, a partner who isn't taking Covid as seriously as you are, an at-risk family member who has decided they "just want to live normally." There may be someone in your life that you really care about who isn't being safe and you just want them to know you're worried.

Being around other Covid-safe people is one of the most relaxing, soul-recharging, and healing things you can do. Nothing compares to spending time with people you know are doing everything they can to avoid Covid. Not having to explain or excuse your masking, having to ask to see people's tests because you don't know if they actually took one, dreading inevitable moments of reminding people that no, you're not able to go inside for lunch. Does your nan complain that you never stay very long? When you're sharing in-person time with other Covid-safe people you don't feel rushed to leave. You can slow down and spend more time because you're jamming with air purifiers blazing and not watching an Aranet4 scream red that you need to get out ASAP.

When you're around other Covid-safe people it's like having a huge weight off your shoulders for the first time in forever. No one is judging you about having Covid boundaries. No one doubts you for avoiding risk. You don't have to worry about how they'll treat you or judge your anecdote about winking at a fellow masker in the DMV the other day, and they'll commiserate with you about the lack of masks on the train. There are entire stressful conversations you don't need to have, like explaining why you don't want Covid. What's more, you know the Covid-safe people you're with are some of the people who still care about themselves, their loved ones, about you, their communities, and our shared future.

Being able to spend time around Covid-safe people is one thing. It's also a huge relief to know that someone you care about is on the same page with Covid-19 risks and safety practices. If mom is masking at the supermarket and your bestie skipped a party where she knew everyone would be hotboxing Covid, then you know they're not only safer for you to be around, but that they're not taking a risk that could have them end up bed bound with Long Covid. And you know they're part of the solution to this mess we're in, not one of the people perpetuating a pandemic.

It's a terrible feeling when an at-risk family member or friend—and let's face it, most everyone is at-risk now if they've had Covid-19 even once—acts like everything is pre-pandemic "back to normal."

It hurts our hearts to see what happened, and is still happening to Dianna Cowern, aka Physics Girl.[1] Cowern was a science communicator for PBS, then went indie. Her one and only Covid-19 infection in June 2022 left her disabled with Long Covid and ME/CFS since then. She's still completely bed-bound, can't speak much, can no longer eat most kinds of food, and uses a bedside urinal. Her husband is her full-time caretaker and works with her care team to raise awareness about Covid-19 risks and Long Covid.[2]

For me, when I think about someone carelessly or unknowingly exposing me to Covid, or hear a risk-taking friend say they don't want to talk about Covid anymore, I always wonder if I need to mentally prepare myself for that friend's life being upended and ways it will change if they become newly and unexpectedly disabled. If it can happen to Dianna Cowern, it can happen to anyone. With ongoing mass infections, it is happening to unsuspecting people every day, including kids, who don't yet realize it.

Either way, the Covid prevention conversation has to happen. Let's look at some potential goals. You might want to:

- Spend more time with someone.
- Be able to attend an event, or a holiday visit.
- Provide accurate, nonjudgemental prevention and risk information.
- Help someone understand what they're risking.
- Help someone understand the risk they pose to you.
- Clear up confusion about transmission and prevention tools.
- Help someone understand your Covid boundaries.
- Repair trust in the relationship.
- Tell someone how to make a gathering safer.
- Encourage masking with the outlook that imperfect masking is better than no masking at all.
- Find out if someone knows that masks have come a long way in five years.
- Help someone get the right masks.
- Help someone practice self-advocacy in the healthcare system.
- Find out why someone stopped masking/trying to prevent infection.
- Find out if someone knows that the virus has changed, and Covid is worse than we thought.
- Help someone understand that avoiding a virus that causes death and disability is not a "mental illness."

Bringing it up can feel scary and the conversation might make you feel vulnerable, anxious, sad, mad, or even defensive. Try to notice what's coming up for you and acknowledge it without judgment. Remind yourself to stay open and listen.

CONVERSATION STARTERS

One option is to use an external prompt to start the conversation. That can come from sharing an article about Covid-19 rampaging at the 2024 Olympics, Physics Girl, a celebrity with Long Covid, a Covid-related cancellation, Violet Affleck's masks, or photos of people in masks behind the scenes in their favorite TV show. Articles from reputable sources relaying new information about Covid, like Covid and diabetes, are good too—just avoid sending someone links to Facebook groups, technical papers, or barraging them with studies. Don't send links to masks or air purifiers until after you know they're open to these ideas.:

- "Did you see that article about Covid at the Olympics?"
- "I'm a big fan of Physics Girl. Did you hear what happened to her?"
- "Have you seen those photos of Violet Affleck?"
- "Wow, I had no idea everyone on the set of *Fallout* was masked. Did you?"
- "What did you think of that *New York Times* article about Long Covid?"

Another option for conversation starters is to ask questions about their point of view. Find out why they feel the way they do about taking precautions, why they stopped masking, why they didn't get a booster shot. Find things you agree with in their responses and establish some common ground.

- "Hey I know this was a while ago but what was the reason you stopped masking?"
- "Do you ever worry about Long Covid?"

- "I'm just curious, is there a reason you're not getting a booster shot?"
- "Avoiding Covid is really important to me, I'm just wondering what your take on it is."

Link Covid risk and prevention with a topic they care about or community they're interested in, or an analogy to something personally familiar. "I've used HIV as an analogy, not to instill fear in people," explained podcaster Misha, "but within queer circles it tends to be very effective because most of us know about condoms and PrEP, and PEP, and retrovirals, and viral load etc. etc. And many of us didn't know what it was like before."[3] Covid is directly affecting pretty much everything right now so there are a range of topics to tie into, like the economy, disability rights, healthcare equity, worker's rights, kids and pregnant people, cancer survivors, musicians and actors, pets and wildlife, women's health issues, and more.

- "Wow, did you see that article on the economic impact of Long Covid in Australia?"
- "You may be interested in a new report about Covid infection during pregnancy, at least as a heads-up."
- "Did you hear about what happened to Morgan Fairchild's fiancee? It's so sad, they were together for 40 years."
- "I'm a bit freaked out about the new info on Covid and cats. Have you seen it?"
- "I can't believe they're not masking at the cancer center."

You can also ask them to help *you* solve the problem of trying to not get infected at an event, or advice on how to ask one of your friends to wear a mask in the car:

- "So I know it's not exactly your thing, but I could really use your advice."
- "You're good at this: how do you think I should ask my roommate to do a Covid test after Burning Man?"
- "Can I get your opinion on something? I'm trying to figure out the best way to ask Fred to wear a mask for our morning commute."
- "I have these tickets to see a play but I'm stressed about the Covid risk. What do you think I should do?"
- "Simone is getting married and I want to go so bad, but at Amy's reception last year *everyone* got Covid. I can't lose my sick days. What do you think I should do?"

Add humor where you can. For instance, if they say something like "I'm not going to mask forever" you can respond with "OMG me neither!" They indicated this is a binary problem and that things may never change, and you responded by acknowledging the absurdity of the issue being binary while agreeing that no, you don't want to have to do this forever either (but we still do for now). Suggest ridiculous situations to break up the tension.

SERVICES AND EVENTS

If leadership had chosen a path of prevention during the first Covid-19 vaccine rollout, that would've included continued masking in both public and private event spaces, air quality upgrades and clean air minimums for indoor spaces, as well as continued and transparent disease surveillance and the timely dissemination of accurate Covid information. I often wonder what things would be like now if that had happened. Instead, the onus was shifted to individuals to fend for ourselves while businesses, venues, and public spaces were left with no guidance, information, or support.

Now we're faced with making hard and sometimes sad decisions about any time we spend indoors or around others. So when we get invited to gatherings, there are Comic-Cons we want to attend, or our best friend decides to throw a party, we can either attend as safely as possible or not go at all. It goes from feeling personally frustrating and stressful to seeming like willful negligence when event organizers and party-throwers damn well know better but choose to ignore Covid safety protocols for all involved.

The reality we're stuck with right now is one where we get invites to parties, work meetings, and gatherings that don't include information on testing, masking, or ventilation, while the same goes for most conferences and businesses. This is both a Covid prevention problem and disability accessibility issue.

In most cases, it won't hurt to ask hosts or service providers what their Covid prevention protocols are before you go. It may feel awkward, and you may get an ignorant answer, but there remains a small chance that someone will make a change that leads to a safer event, even if by a little bit.

This could be in the form of an indoor wedding adding an outdoor space for socializing at the reception. An event that recommends masks or moves from recommendation to requirement. Or an organization adding Covid-19 safety information to its attendee guide. A venue agreeing to provide optional outdoor space for attendees. Or an event that adds mask-required hours (masked mornings in the vendor halls), a masked silent disco event for socializing, gives speakers the option to require masks at their talk, or provides N95 masks and RAT tests on site. A group of people agreeing to wear masks at the meetup and/or agreeing to test beforehand. A testing station at the entrance. You might even inspire someone to add air purifiers to an indoor space.

First, the awkward part. Steel yourself and ask what you need to know about Covid-19 prevention at the event, at the party, or in the dentist's office. There's nothing wrong with advocating for your health and well-being. The thing that's deeply wrong is that we've been made to feel awkward, ashamed, embarrassed, or like a burden for not wanting to get a deadly and disabling virus that could destroy our lives with one wrong breath.

If you really feel nervous about it, ask a buddy or fellow Covid-conscious advocate to make the phone call or send an email for you. Here are some talking point ideas to get you started:

- "Hey, I was just wondering what Covid prevention things you're doing for the event."
- "I can't seem to find any information on your website/in your 'Accessibility' section about Covid safety for attendees/guests. Can you direct me to your Covid policies?"
- "I'm just gathering some pre-event information. How are you making the conference Covid-safe for high-risk attendees?"
- "Hi there, I'm coming in for an appointment next week and need to be very careful about Covid. Will staff wear masks on request?"
- "I really want to do our Tuesday meeting but I can't lose any sick days to Covid. Can we please all wear masks?"
- "Will guests have to test for Covid before the party?"
- "I need to be extra cautious right now. What's your venue's ventilation situation like?"
- "I'd really feel more comfortable if you wore a mask."
- "Are you offering an outdoor area for socializing? We really want to see everybody and it's going to make it easier for us to attend."

- "Thank you for inviting me. I'm not doing indoor events that don't have Covid precautions right now, will there be any masking, testing, or ventilation information available?"

The World Health Network has a very straightforward, detailed guide called "Asking for Safer Precautions."[4] It focuses on two primary strategies that are aligned with escalating the request through legal means, specifically the US American Disabilities Act, with a template suited for contacting specific services, such as a medical provider. WHN explains: "While some organizations and individuals are resistant to helping with safety protections, others may be helpful either due to an adequate appreciation of the risks, or due to respecting the wishes of those making a request... a general recommendation is to approach the beginning of a request by presenting a clear discussion of a set of options that you would like to see implemented, acknowledging that some of them may not be possible." They suggest having a list of areas to address based on the 5 pillars of protection: "Respirator masks, Ventilation and HEPA filtration, Testing, Distancing, Vaccination."

> *"I see about 150-200 patients a week, many of them with hoarking coughs, right in my face. And I didn't catch a single thing from them. Masks in health care settings is just common sense."* —Kashif Pirzada, MD

In her explainer *How To Stay Covid Safe When In Hospital*, The Disabled Ginger wrote: "Speak to the staff at the hospital and see if you can come to an arrangement where healthcare workers who are treating you will be required to mask... if possible ask to speak to a nurse floor manager or a patient relations representative, explain your concerns and offer to provide masks if they don't have any. Consider placing a sign on the door that says 'Masks Required for Entry' along with spare masks."[5]

Healthcare settings are one of the most dangerous places for anyone to be right now. They have always been dangerous and potentially deadly for disabled, immunocompromised, and chronically ill people (yes, that includes Long Covid), but now they're extremely high-risk–it's gotten deadly *and* deadlier. Anti-masking attitudes and policies are widespread in hospitals, treatment centers, and doctor's offices around the world. The false belief that Covid-19 is benign, infection is harmless or "builds immunity," or any of the prevalent Covid myths create horror-movie healthcare scenarios for immunocompromised and at-risk people, particularly BIPOC, LGBTQIA+, disabled people, and women. An enormous number of people are forced to determine whether it's riskier to get essential medical care and potentially get infected, or leave their illness or injury untreated.

Learn more about Covid-19 and medical gaslighting in the chapter, "Long Covid And Relationships." These targeted groups need our advocacy and support. Read how to take what we've learned in this chapter and become an effective advocate for high-risk patients in the chapter "Make Anger Useful."

DIFFICULT OUTCOMES

You'll be met with misinformation a lot: most people are deeply uninformed about Covid-19 right now—it's not their fault. Don't tell them they're wrong about something outright; this will send their defenses up. If they insist on incorrect facts try to tell them how you feel ("I'm scared of Long Covid") and stories about your friends

("Michelle has Long Covid so bad right now, I miss seeing her so much").

During your conversations, you may encounter some pretty wild misconceptions or beliefs, such as someone saying masks don't work, masks limit oxygen intake, or that masks have chemicals that make people sick—or even completely false conspiracy theories like vaccines causing autism, causing Long Covid, or carrying microchips.

One of my hobbies is gaming. In the first year of the pandemic I was in the United States, in San Francisco, California. While we sheltered in place I spent a lot of time in online games. I'd often join teams or form pairs with people I didn't know who were located all over the world, and spent many hours doing quests while talking to strangers through my headphones. I got to meet all kinds of gamers who were all experiencing the first year of Covid-19 in ways much different than mine and I learned a lot. Some of it was interesting, like that firefighters in Oregon were code-naming their Covid-19 calls "Charlie" (or "possible Charlie").

I also met a lot of young gamer dudes who believed some pretty outlandish stuff about Covid. It was all conspiracy theories they'd learned from adults in Facebook or Telegram groups, though almost every single time I asked them where they heard that, or where they got their news about Covid-19, they would answer "Facebook." When I would ask why they didn't get news from actual news sources, they would ask me how to do that, and where I was getting my news. They didn't know where to get accurate information.

As you can imagine, I heard some wild conspiracies stated as fact. Because they were young adults I knew that they were essentially "trying out" the statements on me to see if they would be validated or not, or get a reaction of some kind. So when someone I'd been raiding nuclear silos with in *Fallout* for hours would say "I'm not getting the vaccine. Because, you know. *Microchips*." This actually happened several times. I would always explode in laughter and say, "Seriously?"

Next, I ask where their information came from (always Facebook), because I could always get them to laugh at Facebook as a great news source if you have brain worms, or BNN (Boomer News Nightly). My main aim was getting them to see how completely hilarious the conspiracy belief was by discussing practicalities. Like talking about how expensive all those microchips would be, and even if everyone was "chipped" it would be broken like everything tech is right now anyway. Breaking down how the conspiracy theory would actually work in real life (poorly, expensively) inevitably led to the conspiracy's underlying fear, which is fear of control, tracking, and surveillance. At which point I'd say: "Bro—your *phone* is a tracking device." Because there's no need for a microchip when they've already chipped themselves, I'd point out.

If anything, their Facebook app was "chipping" them. This was always followed by a moment of silence. I wasn't "debating" anyone, a tactic which makes people dig their heels in deeper and helps them rehearse their arguments. I was talking to young people trying to make sense of the world who were dealing with rotten adults in places where they had no one else to talk to.

Britannica describes conspiracy theories as "an attempt to explain harmful or tragic events as the result of the actions of a small powerful group. Such explanations reject the accepted narrative surrounding those events; indeed, the official version may be seen as further proof of the conspiracy... Conspiracy theories increase in prevalence in periods of widespread anxiety, uncertainty, or hardship, as during wars and economic depressions and in the aftermath of natural disasters like tsunamis, earthquakes, and pandemics."[6] Britannica adds: "Conspiratorial thinking is driven by a strong human desire to make sense of social forces that are self-relevant, important, and threatening." Many Covid-19 conspiracy theories come from far-right ideologies and are used to sow division, undermine trust in institutions, are used to demonize groups of people by fueling racial hatred and eugenicist discrimination against disabled people. Covid conspiracy disinformation is usually interwoven in conspiracy beliefs of people motivated to violence.

When a friend or loved one believes Covid conspiracies, you might feel motivated to debunk them on the spot, or send them a flurry of articles and studies to try and get them back into a Covid safety, science-forward prevention mindset. However, confrontational debunking, even with facts, seldom works—when faced with information that counters their beliefs, the believer will usually double-down. That's because, per Britannica, conspiracy believers engage in "biased assimilation, whereby information that supports one's position is uncritically accepted, whereas contrary information is scrutinized and discredited. Further, because of attitude polarization, when people encounter ambiguous information, they tend to endorse their original position even more strongly than they did prior to encountering the information."

A more effective strategy is to "pre-bunk" conspiracy theories. This is when you warn someone about bad information before it has a chance to take root or grow. Great pre-bunking tools for sharing include *Bad News* (getbadnews.com),[7] an online disinformation media literacy game, the World Health Organization's Covid-19 misinformation literacy game *Go Viral!* (goviralgame.com),[9] and DebunkBot,[8] an AI chatbot from MIT that's been shown to reduce conspiratorial beliefs by 20%.[10]

In the "References and Resources" chapter you'll find a range of tools and approaches to help you try and pull a friend or family member out of it. In summary, primary advice consists of learning more about their conspiracy theories, avoiding telling them they're wrong, encouraging critical thinking, prioritizing their health if possible, and not writing them off completely.

Since we're talking about Covid-19 safety and prevention, you may need to make difficult choices about the Covid risk (or threat) this person poses to you and people you care about. Cutting ties or taking extended "time off" are valid self-preservation options. As anyone who has encountered substance abuse therapy will tell you, if someone doesn't want to "be there" it's pretty much impossible to change their behavior.

My encounters debunking gamer buddies were all conversations that could've gone very badly and I'm glad to say I made a lot of new pals who got vaccinated. Sadly, conversations about Covid with friends, loved ones, and family members who have adopted conspiracy theory beliefs don't often go as well. Asking someone with strongly held conspiracy beliefs why they believe something or where they got their information can cause reactions of defensiveness, anger, aggression, meanness or cruelty, emotional manipulation, gaslighting, and other forms of abuse.

"There's also a phenomenon of displaced anger from some people that haven't worked through the trauma of the last 3 years," explained Dr. Lisa Iannattone in a Twitter thread. "They weirdly direct their anger about the pandemic at me, as if I'm Covid, instead of working through their feelings about the pandemic in a healthy way. I've literally had to stop people to say 'Hey, it sounds like you're upset about how Covid changed a lot of things, but you seem to be directing your anger at me? I'm not the virus. None of this is even remotely my fault and I can't fix it for you.'"

Unless you are a trained therapist or counselor, you're quite literally not equipped to deal with this problem, nor do you have the training to keep yourself safe from vitriol, attacks, or abuse. Try to remember that this person is struggling with fear and anger, especially because the realities of Covid and being abandoned by leadership in a deadly and disabling ongoing pandemic are too terrifying for some people to cope with. This is understandable, but staying safe in *every* way is your top priority. If you are determined to reach this person, get guidance from a therapist or counselor every step of the way.

It's okay to take a break from the relationship or friendship. If you need to take extended time off from them that's okay, too–though consider holding space for them in the future should they reconsider their beliefs. Think of it like someone leaving a cult. People who walk away from conspiracy groups wind up ostracized and socially rejected by people in those groups, and typically face the prospect of having few friends or family to turn to when they hope to rebuild their lives.

REMAIN OPEN

Expect this discussion to develop over time. This is not going to be a one-time conversation. It's ongoing: slow and steady wins the race. You're probably not going to convince mom to mask up for grocery shopping overnight, or turn her weekly indoor lunches into weekly outside walks. You're making space for her to move into and encouraging her to reduce risk and harms. She may mask indoors but forget a few crucial details, and it doesn't mean you failed. It means she's trying. She may mask for a while and then stop—but if you make space for her to start again, she might find it easier to do so.

Listen, listen, listen: don't lecture. Avoid using jargon, social justice terminology that might be off-putting, or referring to deeply technical details. Meet them where they are with language. Most people don't understand air quality readings and wastewater data, let alone how to use them, and that's okay—but people tend to shut off when a topic becomes too complicated. Remember that what you're explaining is really scary. Also, no one wants to be told that what they know or something they believe is inaccurate or false.

You may need to repeat information you've explained before. Try to do so without reminding them you've covered this ground previously. It may not have sunk in for them last time, and our brains tend to edit out things we don't get or find complicated, or unpleasant. Rally fresh energy to explain why masks need to be airtight or why the virus loves stale air like it's the first time, and your audience will be more receptive to hearing about it.

COVID GASLIGHTING

> "When one asks for the minimum protections, even the most sensible individuals shrug and say, 'but for how long?' Covid has yielded the most stunningly pervasive gaslighting phenomenon in recent history." —Tithi Bhattacharya, Truthout[1]

SOME MIGHT THINK GASLIGHTING is something that only happens in abusive intimate relationships. Yet the ongoing pandemic shows us gaslighting can happen in any circumstance, from friends, coworkers, and family members to public health institutions, characterization of illness, headlines, political maneuvers, PR messaging, data manipulation, and more.

Gaslighting is a nearly 100-year-old term that's become increasingly popular in the past few years due to wider societal interest in mental health, primarily through social media. It comes from a play (made into the film "Gaslight") in which a woman notices the gas-fuel lights in her house occasionally dim; her husband convinces her it's not happening by making her believe it's all in her head. In truth, the lights flicker when he goes into the attic to steal from her. Gaslighters can be any gender, and systemic gaslighting is also a mechanism, though most gaslighting targets tend to be women, disabled people, BIPOC, and marginalized communities; racism, ageism, and sizeism are also factors.

Gaslighters rewrite history, discredit you, distract you, shift blame, minimize your feelings, and lie to you. Gaslighting is an abuse technique that undermines our perception of reality and isolates us. It's a tool for controlling someone's behavior by making you second-guess yourself, your risk calculations, your memories, recent events, and your perceptions.

When someone gaslights you, they try to convince you that their experience of things is the real one, and yours is not. Like that everyone but you is "back to normal" despite rolling waves of sickness and escalating Long Covid disability. A gaslighter will sow self-doubt, confusion, and isolation, such as when someone responds to an inquiry about Covid protections at a wedding by saying "no one does that anymore." They'll tell you you're overreacting to or misinterpreting Covid's risk despite an abundance of well-documented, sometimes deathly serious post-infection conditions. A gaslighter will tell you you're remembering things wrong, bully you into conforming to their risk model, or play their abuse about your masking as "just a joke," and make you question your reality.

Gaslighting can make you feel like you're "too sensitive" or overreacting, despite the gravity and seriousness of your concerns. You might feel afraid of speaking up because you doubt yourself, or like trying to convince yourself that something isn't "that bad." Gaslighting makes you doubt yourself and your decisions; it hammers your self-esteem and heightens feelings of insecurity. It also makes you feel isolated because you're being convinced that you're "crazy" or "hysterical.. Gaslighting hinges on making you feel powerless and alone.

Gaslighting harms our mental state if it goes unrecognized and unexamined. According to the Newport Institute, "People who experience gaslighting are at a high risk for anxiety, depression, and suicidal thoughts."[2] Covid gaslighting ups the stakes by making us doubt our judgement and trust in ourselves in the face of risking a deadly and disabling disease. It can upend worldviews we hold about people being generally good and trust in healthcare systems. It can feel soul-destroying to see article after article from major news outlets contorting themselves into pretzels to avoid saying the word "Covid" and the brain-breaking illogic of insisting on referring to Covid in the past tense—even in reports about surges and outbreaks.

One of gaslighting's key mechanisms is minimizing—that's the opposite of exaggeration. This is a type of deception that blends denial with rationalization in situations where blanket denial clearly won't work. Like downplaying Covid-19 severity by saying anyone not hospitalized had a "mild" case, discounting the degree of disability that comes with Long Covid, invalidating Long Covid risk by associating it with preexisting conditions, dismissing concerns about risk by comparing it to a cold, or being told you're the only one who still cares about Covid. This can also be telling you they "had it worse," renaming things like Covid-19 deaths as "died with" versus "died of" to downplay Covid as the cause or contributing factor, or downplaying the efficacy of masks.

In every instance of gaslighting as described by mental health organizations, counselors, and therapists, gaslighting is very clearly defined as abuse. The standard advice for someone who is in a relationship where they are being gaslighted is to get out. The Newport Institute explained, "Once you've figured out how to tell if someone is gaslighting you, the next step is removing yourself from the relationship, if at all possible, and avoiding other potential gaslighting situations." Ending a relationship is terrible, and always easier said than done.

But what do we do when the gaslighting is actually a public health emergency?

Covid gaslighting is a tool for convincing people Covid is benign and to discourage prevention. If someone tells you "the pandemic is over" or refers to Covid-19 in the past-tense, especially while you are still there with a mask on your face, you are being gaslit.

There are three ways we're experiencing Covid gaslighting. In order to better protect ourselves from its harms, understand how to heal from it, and build resiliency, let's examine what's going on.

One way we experience Covid gaslighting is in face-to-face interactions. That can come from friends, loved ones, family members, or coworkers, and people who have power over us, such as a boss, client, teacher, landlord, driver, doctor, security guard, and law enforcement.

The second type of Covid gaslighting we encounter is situational. This can be an event, wedding, hospital or healthcare setting, and settings that discourage or prohibit masks.

The third way we're experiencing Covid gaslighting is from politics and media, including political messaging and decision-making, headlines and articles, and the entertainment industry, through film and TV. It is disinformation: presenting false information about Covid-19 or prevention tools to control or change your behavior.

FACE-TO-FACE COVID GASLIGHTING

Face-to-face Covid gaslighting is a type of abuse. Even if you can't stop it or walk away, it's important to recognize that it's happening. Here are Covid gaslighting phrases you may recognize, placed within the "5 types of gaslighting" framework:

Manipulation of reality
You're overreacting.
Why do you have to make a big deal about it?
You sound paranoid.
You're living in fear.
Why can't you move on?
Everyone is living normally except you.
Stop being hysterical.

Trivializing (minimizing)
It's like the flu.
I've had it, it's not a big deal/it's milder.
I used to mask and I got it anyway.
It was never that bad.
John had it three times and he's fine.
Kids don't get it that bad.
Long Covid isn't that common.
Infectious diseases have existed forever, worse ones than Covid.

Scapegoating
It's a pandemic of the unvaccinated.
Healthy people don't have to worry.
Only people with preexisting conditions get Long Covid.
Those tests don't always work.
Only vulnerable people are at risk.

Lying (including disinformation and misinformation)
We need to get exposed so we build immunity.
It's just like a cold now.
No one masks anymore.
We've all moved on.
Covid is mild now.
Kids don't get it.
Reinfections are rare.
Masks don't work.

Coercion
No one else is masking.
Are you going to wear a mask forever?
I can't live like that (or "no one" can).
I can't hear you [in that mask].
You can't avoid it forever.
But the CDC says...
You just need to deal with it.
But doctors aren't wearing masks.
We have to live with Covid.
It is time to move on.

IDENTIFY, ASSESS, ACT

When you are being gaslit, the best advice is to name it—recognize you are being gaslit in that moment—and change direction. Identify the gaslighting, assess the risks, and decide how to proceed.

Don't let someone make you doubt your Covid boundaries, and never change a boundary or break one of your Covid rules in the heat of the moment. *Psychology Today* explains, "Gaslighting isn't about a misunderstanding; it's a psychological tactic to undermine your sense of reality. We have to completely disengage from the pull to defend ourselves and instead show that we are confident in our memory of events well enough that we don't need them to believe us. We believe us, and that is enough."[3]

Ask yourself if the wedding, conference, work meeting, family dinner, feeling like you don't fit in for one hour, makeout session or sex, visit to the hairdresser, night at the bar, or lunch with your best friend will be worth having Long Covid. Or worth the possibility that you end up being one of the people who has to crawl to the bathroom on all fours most days. If you really doubt a Covid boundary you've made, wait until later to think about deciding to change it.

Size up the situation. A family member telling you to "stop living in fear" by wearing a mask may or may not understand they're being abusive. It's most likely that if you tell them what they are doing in the moment and that it's abusive behavior, they may not react well or be receptive to this information. Few people know how to handle being told they're hurting someone, nor do most people have the tools to deal well with being told they're wrong.

Oftentimes you may opt to ignore a gaslighting statement, and that's perfectly okay. Deciding not to act is still your decision to make. No one who threatens your Covid boundaries deserves your energy. You can simply shrug and move on to another subject, and decide what to do about it later, if anything.

You can opt to respond by making a boundary, and there are many techniques and several sample phrases for Covid boundary setting in the chapter "Covid Boundaries." These responses can offer easy rebuffs to gaslighters or give you an "out" when someone is gaslighting by coercion. Keep in mind that gaslighters often get hostile when their tactic doesn't work. If it's someone you care about, one option is to exit the conversation and pick it up later as a talking point to see if you can get them a bit more informed about Covid and your point of view.

Responding to Covid gaslighting when it's outright lying is a judgment call you may need to make in the moment. Ask yourself if it's worth disagreeing with this person. Consider whether they might escalate to hostility or use gaslighting comments designed to hurt you. Keeping yourself safe in every way is your top priority. If it's someone you have the energy and time to educate about misinformation, then buckle in—and refer to the chapter "Talking About Covid" for debunking and "pre bunking" techniques.

More than anything, social or interpersonal Covid gaslighting comes from a place of fear. Fear of Covid's realities, of being wrong, of being humiliated, of feeling out of control or losing control, fear that comes with helplessness, fear of loss, and being afraid of an uncertain future. We feel these things, too. The difference is that we've learned how to make fear into a productive response of practical prevention, risk assessment, and community care. Not one of denial, risk-taking, or manipulation.

SITUATIONAL COVID GASLIGHTING

You probably noticed that many Covid gaslighting phrases in the previous section are also commonly-held, widespread myths about Covid-19. They're easily disproved with years of verified data and thousands of reputable studies—but the myths persist and are widely considered to be fact. That's because we're living through a massive public health failure at scale.

Situational Covid gaslighting is when gaslighting is part of the fabric: in systems or the organizing of events, such as when an organization engages in Covid gaslighting. This is when an event or setting should be doing appropriate infection control and masking, or offer options, or afford Covid-safe access, and refuses, dismisses, or ignores the problem.

Examples include:

• Exhortations to "be kind to mask wearers."
• Pretending there's nothing they can do about Covid.
• No masking requirements in hospitals and healthcare settings.
• Weddings and birthday parties with no outdoor areas for socializing.
• Events that ignore the need for, prohibit, or discourage masking.
• Indoor events that ignore air quality concerns or Covid AQ minimums.
• Knowing you mask and inviting you to an indoor dinner party.
• Conferences with no online option.
• Flight attendants prohibiting portable air purifiers.
• Events that respond to Covid prevention inquiries by discouraging your attendance.
• Event materials that offer hand washing as Covid prevention.
• Reduced workplace sick time for Covid; forcing employees to work because "it's just a cold now."
• Healthcare workers saying they are not required to mask.
• Responses to Covid safety questions that offer hand sanitizer (Paris 2024 Olympics).
• Responses to event Covid safety and accessibility questions or re-

quests that frame masking or prevention tools as a personal choice.
• Doctors or nurses characterize a patient as having "anxiety" for requesting masks.
• Events that use "post pandemic" phrasing in information about accessibility.

In March 2023 we learned that over 10% of people who'd caught Covid-19 in Australian hospitals had died from it.[4] So you'd think that at this point in the pandemic, hospitals would require masking, full stop. And with the regular reports of conferences acting as superspreaders—including hundreds of infected at the US CDC's 2023 Epidemic Intelligence Service (EIS) Conference[5]—these events should take all necessary steps to protect attendees from Covid as much as possible. But they're not, and a lot of people who don't want Covid have considered conferences and healthcare too great a Covid risk for several years.

Covid gaslighting we encounter in this context is both situational and systemic. Belgian inclusivity workplace consultancy 3Plus explains: "Systemic gaslighting involves the pervasive use of language within institutions, media, and wider cultures to distort reality, obscure the truth, and control narratives. This can manifest in various forms, from the softer nuances to the more overt."[6] They add, "Within social institutions, language can be wielded to perpetuate harmful norms and maintain power structures. Discriminatory policies may be disguised in bureaucratic jargon, and systems protected by euphemistic and misleading language."

Covid gaslighting is weaponized in systemic gaslighting for reinforcing racial gaslighting, LGBTQIA+, and disability gaslighting. Disability gaslighting is understood through the lens of ableism. "Ableism is the discrimination of and social prejudice against people with disabilities based on the belief that typical abilities are superior," as described by U Cincinnati.[7] "At its heart, ableism is rooted in the assumption that disabled people require 'fixing' and defines people by their disability. Like racism and sexism, ableism classifies entire groups of people as 'less than,' and includes harmful stereotypes, misconceptions, and generalizations of people with disabilities."

Systemic gaslighting weaponizes Covid gaslighting against disabled people through lack of compliance with disability rights laws, refusal to accommodate (like a healthcare setting or nurse refusing to mask), and eugenicist attitudes (or practices) toward the value of disabled lives in an ongoing pandemic. This includes a January 2022 national television appearance where CDC Director Rochelle Walensky said it was "really encouraging" that the Omicron variant was predominantly killing Americans who had "other health problems."[8] Monstrous? Completely.

It's well-documented that women, BIPOC, queer people, and disabled people are more likely to have their symptoms and requests dismissed by medical professionals. This is also called medical gaslighting. Medical gaslighting with all aspects of Covid-19 (transmission, prevention, risk, symptoms, treatment, post-Covid fallout) has reached surreal levels. Against a backdrop of Covid gaslighting, racial gaslighting in healthcare escalates the dual public health crises of Covid and racism.[9] It compounds situations where people of color already face healthcare professionals that continuously dispute medical facts and the patient's personal experience.[10] This leaves patients untreated or undertreated, characterizing them as drug-seekers, disbelieving symptoms, avoiding Long Covid as a diagnosis, being forced to avoid demanding better care (or "remain calm").[11]

To understand more about medical gaslighting and Covid-19, particularly how it's weaponized and disproportionately targeting disabled, chronically ill, people of color and women who are hardest-hit by the pandemic, queer people, and very notably people and kids who have Long Covid, skip ahead to the chapter "Long Covid And Relationships."

SOCIETAL AND POLITICAL COVID GASLIGHTING

In *London Review of Books*, author Christienna Fryar examined the book *Age of Emergency: Living with Violence at the End of the British Empire* by Erik Linstrum.[12] The book describes how there became two prevailing versions about the way the British Empire ended as described by official language and media, especially news outlets.

One was that the end of the British Empire was a decisive and neat disbanding, a benevolent granting of independence to the colonies.

This is something US readers of this book will recognize in much the same way as the Biden Administration's White House "ended" the Covid-19 pandemic by merely saying it was "over," cutting all emergency and prevention services, and nearly eliminated public data sharing, virus surveillance, and tracking of cases. This was kicked off by a White House event on July 4, 2021, branded and messaged in a speech by President Biden titled "Celebrating Independence Day and Independence from COVID-19."[13]

The second version of the British Empire's end, per Fryar, "claims that the end of empire was in fact extremely violent, but that knowledge of this violence was successfully suppressed, both at the time and in the decades since." Fryar adds, "There was a careful dance between keeping the worst details quiet while allowing the right kind of information to get out, in the hope that the public would accept some brutality as the price of securing Britain's place in the world."

By official counts—which are well-documented and widely acknowledged as undercounts—nearly one million Americans (and counting) have died from Covid-19 since July 4, 2021, and at least 17 million (and counting) in the US are living with becoming newly disabled by Long Covid.[14] To this day, wave after wave every 3-4 months mass infects the population with a new strain of the virus whose aftereffects we are only beginning to understand and include diabetes, heart damage and disease, cognitive effects and new onset dementia, POTS, and a list of severe conditions too long to include here.

Nearly five years of children have been born during this time of repeated mass infection in the US, a significant number of which now have new-onset diabetes, heart conditions, and Long Covid—estimated at 6 million and counting.[15] Per Kaiser Family Foundation (2022), "Total cumulative data show Black, Hispanic, American Indian or Alaska Native (AIAN), and Native Hawaiian or Other Pacific Islander (NHOPI) people have experienced higher rates of Covid-19 cases and deaths compared to White people."[16]

It would appear that "Independence from Covid-19" is a conspicuously white affair. And despite the official language, the unthinkable US Covid death count climbs every week with the prospect of tens of millions newly disabled, spanning generations to come, sitting on its doorstep growing steadily, unable to just "go away."

Most countries around the world followed the US playbook, such as the UK's similarly-timed "Freedom Day" on July 19, 2021—itself contradicted in real time by soaring cases of the Delta variant.[17] The US led the world in dismantling the public health response to the pandemic largely by combining policy changes and announcements with coordinated messaging, which is historically how these things are done.

The clearest examples of this were essentially coordinated gaslighting; anti-prevention or Covid minimizing claims to bolster public perceptions made in concert between top US news outlets and White House officials. One instance was in July 2023, in a *New York Times* piece stating US Covid death numbers were "an exaggeration."[18] The article quoted the White House Covid Coordinator, Ashish Jha, and then was promoted by him in his official capacity on social media channels.

Other news outlets and organizations participated in the official cultivation of public acceptance for Covid-19's ongoing, mounting sickness, disability, and death. But *The New York Times* played a crucial part in September 2021, when many of us were seeing and experiencing Covid reinfections, and the White House rushed to gaslight the existence of reinfections altogether.

On September 7, *NYT* unequivocally stated: "One in 5,000: The real chances of a breakthrough infection."[19] The article added, "It's not clear how much we should be worrying about them." Interestingly, that "One in 5,000" claim cited data from Utah, Virginia, and Washington—when no data was available. In fact, the *Virginia Mercury* reported on August 27, 2021 that the Virginia Department of Health "isn't reporting the percentage of breakthrough cases out of all total known infections week-by-week."[20]

Nonetheless, in prepared remarks on September 9, 2021, President Biden stated: "Recent data indicates there is only one confirmed positive case per 5,000 fully vaccinated Americans per day."[21] The "no breakthroughs" fallacy was followed on December 17 2021, when the White House issued a briefing stating Omicron "cases are milder."[22] This was followed by a January 5, 2022, *New York Times* headline stating: "Omicron Is Milder."[23]

There's no conspiracy here: it's coordinated messaging. Yet this is when political gaslighting constitutes a public health emergency, one that has normalized news outlets in discouraging support for prevention tools and practices. *The Atlantic's* May 2021 article "The Liberals Who Can't Quit Lockdown" comes to mind.[24] (The United States never had lockdowns: 3/4 of the country had varying interpretations of "Shelter in Place," "Safer at Home," or "Stay Home" orders.[25]) This coordinated messaging has also normalized the pandemic essentially being edited out of news, opinion media, and entertainment.

You would think that the mounting evidence about Covid's danger—such as mild cases severely infecting and damaging heart muscles—its ongoing, mounting harm—billions of dollars in workforce losses yearly—as well as the increasing millions and millions of people with Long Covid (including children)—horrific, *random* cases of giant populations who lose their freedom/autonomy and ability to function—would change the messaging and reporting around Covid-19 risk and prevention. This duality of perception, one of Covid as tidily past-tense and the other as a daily random risk of potentially horrific lifelong disability for everyone, has a historical precedent in the two different versions of the ending of the British Empire.

"Liberal writers and organisations had far more influence, but were rarely supportive of decolonisation," wrote Christienna Fryar in *London Review of Books*. "Even when they sought to express concern, their statements often ended up bolstering counterinsurgency campaigns. The professional norms and modes of argument they observed demanded deference, deliberation and what was considered objectivity."

Fryar notes that social class, whiteness, a false sense of impartiality, and unwillingness to believe terrible things are happening were key reasons for the myth-making. "This dynamic was perhaps most apparent in newspaper journalism. A *Times* correspondent, Oliver Woods, received a number of reports—including from other journalists and officials—that British soldiers were using torture in Kenya. Yet none of these made their way into his stories, apparently because he was unwilling to believe them. Censorship sometimes came from editors who considered official sources to be more reliable than eyewitness testimony. *The Observer* sat on a dispatch from Kenya for months, then published a heavily edited version that omitted references to violence."

It seems like the same biases are affecting talking heads, politicians, and the systemic Covid-19 gaslighting we're living through right now. Which brings us to one of the more bizarre aspects of Covid gaslighting: pro-infection messaging. We've all seen articles about mildness and statements from pundits saying infections are good for kids, outlets promoting flawed and discredited anti-mask "studies," uncritically repeated talking points about hand washing, the insidious herd immunity myth on repeat, attacks on people who still mask, and so on.

The insistence in perpetuating Covid-19 gaslighting in media also comes from a strong fear of humiliation—the person wielding influence who can't handle being wrong. Which would be a curiosity if it were merely about something mundane, like how shampoo is made, as opposed to critical public health information, like *NYT*'s star Covid pundit David Leonhardt doing high-profile interviews saying that masks aren't very effective against Covid.[26]

COVID GASLIGHTING IN ENTERTAINMENT

There is a strong element throughout "back to normal" gaslighting that firmly places the victims of Covid-19 and the millions of people experiencing an ongoing pandemic outside the discussion.

Nowhere is that more evident than Hollywood, which is still partying—on camera, at least—like it's 2019. Viewers are always surprised to find out that entire movie and television productions, especially crew, still have careful Covid safety rules. Watch behind the scenes clips from HBO's *The Last of Us* or *Our Flag Means Death*, Paramount's *Star Trek: Picard* or *Strange New Worlds*, Netflix's *Bridgerton*, or Amazon Prime's shows *Fallout* and *Evil*. Proper N95 masking on everyone when the cameras aren't rolling, and at all times on crew members—while on outdoor film and TV sets as well. Even making-of video showing orchestral scoring for the animated *Star Trek: Lower Decks* series shows every musician masked while playing cellos, violins, and more–basically, every instrument that wasn't brass or woodwind.

You wouldn't know it because according to the dominant narrative of film and TV over the past three years, Covid-19 never happened and is still not happening, despite a global death toll estimated by *The Economist* to be as high as 35.2 million "With 95% confidence interval" (2022).[27] It takes a lot of work to keep the largest ongoing global pandemic in 100 years absent from nearly every film and TV show purporting to be "modern day."

During that first Covid summer when the US averaged over 1,000 dying a day and refrigerated morgue trucks in major cities were no longer a new concept, we became aware that our serials, talk shows, dramas, sitcoms, reality series, and movies—ones not set in the far future or distant past—seemed like alien time capsules from a previous era. Specifically, 2019. We wondered what would come next, when presumably the world wouldn't end and our shows would create new seasons. We hungered for how our lives, now changed forever, would be reflected.

Covid's US death toll climbed to over 3,000 a day in January 2021; the total death toll for 9/11 was 2,996 Americans. At that time, Hollywood was contorting itself behind the scenes to prevent and avoid Covid in productions as well as award events. Yet simultaneously it became evident that Hollywood was very conspicuously erasing one of the greatest humanitarian crises of the twenty-first century from all dominant film, TV, and pop culture narratives. It's beyond conspicuous now how few movies and shows acknowledge the pandemic, past or present. Some media even makes it worse by minimizing the incredible amount of death we've waded through to get to this point.

Our collective memories are what give us historical consciousness. We currently have next to nothing we can point to and say: this happened, it is still happening, here is what we've lost, and here's why this must never happen again. The Council on Foreign Relations recommends seven (among many) films to help collectively cope with the loss of 2,996 people, to find closure, the value of connection in dark times, understanding the consequences, and to process grief and sadness. But what about when there's at least one 9/11 a week for over three years... while film and TV's dominant narratives erase and seem to actively encourage it? The US had decades of patriotic film and TV focusing on the remembrance of three thousand lives lost on September 11, 2001.

We watch movies and TV to escape, but we need them to reflect our humanity. Actors, film and TV makers, and content creators have been perpetuating a fantasy for nearly three years that there is no pandemic. No "present day" shows or films acknowledge the real present day. By pretending in real life there is no pandemic in films and TV, no public health crisis affecting every corner of everyone's lives, no massive global event disabling our friends, putting our grandparents in coffins, and making our babies sick, we are being denied our ongoing collective experience. We're being gaslit and mocked by the very people we're looking to for some relief in all of this.

We're being robbed of our collective grief.

LONG COVID AND RELATIONSHIPS

> *"I had so many dreams. I wanted my own science show on Netflix. I wanted to start a family with Kyle. I wanted to scuba in Australia. Now, I just want to walk again. I want to have a real conversation. I want to read a book again. I want to listen to music and see my family."* —Dianna Cowern, aka Physics Girl

THE ONLY COVID-19 MEASUREMENTS considered legitimate enough to warrant concern about the virus have been deaths, hospitalizations, and when they become inconvenient, cases. The fact that people weren't recovering—and still aren't—has never been a metric of the pandemic.

The first incidence of Long Covid was reported in 2020, followed by many more.[1] After that, the subsequent use of the #LongCovid hashtag by Dr. Elisa Perego cemented the patient-named condition in public consciousness, we've learned more about it.[2] A large 2024 *Nature Medicine* study showed that 90% of the Covid infections that transition into Long Covid were characterized as "mild."[3] That same study concluded that 400 million people of all ages, genders, and backgrounds around the world have had Long Covid, including people who used to be athletes, kids who didn't have preexisting conditions, famous actors, teachers, politicians, and everyone in between.

We still don't know exactly what causes Long Covid, we don't have a way to prevent it yet (except not getting Covid-19 in the first place), and as of this writing there is still no cure or treatment. Vaccination and timely booster shots can reduce but not eliminate Long Covid risk, which increases with each reinfection.[4]

Long Covid is a constellation of long-term health effects caused by a Covid infection.[5] It is a condition that can affect every system in the body.[6] Long Covid symptoms are often debilitating and can include fatigue or brain fog, ongoing respiratory problems, heart disease, diabetes, neurological problems like cognitive impairment, Postural Orthostatic Tachycardia Syndrome (POTS), and Myalgic Encephalomyelitis/Chronic Fatigue Syndrome (ME/CFS), among others.[7] Some of these conditions are known to be lifelong.

Long Covid is the most researched health condition in any four years of recorded human history (with over 24,000 scientific papers).[8] Despite this, there are a whole lot of people who don't want to acknowledge Long Covid, who refuse to believe it's real, or who adhere to the thinking that Long Covid's scary facts simply can't be true.

The denial and disbelief surrounding Long Covid is pervasive, making its way into media narratives and healthcare settings, workplaces and relationships.[9] As we'd expect, Long Covid denial and disbelief makes everything harder for people who have it, doctors and researchers who want to fight, prevent and treat it, and those whose loved ones have Long Covid. Also—unknowingly—for people who have Long Covid and don't realize it or are unwilling to admit it. We should expect that a lot of people don't know they have Long Covid.

Some people in relationship or family situations where their partner, child, or parent has Long Covid unexpectedly find themselves transitioning into the role of carer. Others may be on the opposite side of that scenario, where they themselves have Long Covid and now rely on a partner or family member struggling to understand or accept the carer role, and in some terrible instances, refusing that role.

Each person who finds themselves in a Long Covid relationship, or even friendship, feels a sense of helplessness and loss. Few people know what to do at first or where to even begin, many struggle with wondering how long this situation will last in its current form, and how this has changed their relationships. It's worse if someone doesn't think Long Covid is real, doesn't think another person's symptoms are real, won't accept that Covid infections can cause potentially permanent disability, or is unwilling to accept that they or a loved one actually has Long Covid.

If any of this sounds familiar: you are not alone. Millions of people are going through these exact scenarios, too. Until recently there were only a handful of community-created resources and few guides; you'll find a wealth of tools and information on long covid in the "References and Resources" chapter.

This chapter is where we explore navigating physical and emotional storms that come with Long Covid and get a better idea about how Long Covid affects our friendships and relationships. This chapter is also designed for handing to a friend or loved one to help them understand something you don't know how to put into words.[10] The sections below can be used as conversation starters when you're not sure how to bring something up. You can also find starting points and sample dialogue in the chapter "Talking About Covid."

WHAT WE WISH EVERYONE KNEW ABOUT LONG COVID

While Long Covid may be one of the most studied conditions in the shortest amount of time ever, it's alarming just how few people know about it. It's astonishing how little of Long Covid's facts and information have made their way into public awareness—or the awareness of medical institutions. This is a disabling disease affecting tens of millions (that we know of), contracted as simply as inhaling bad air, and it's still seldom, if ever, mentioned as a reason to avoid Covid infections. It's the role of public health institutions, their leadership, and healthcare workers everywhere to warn everyone and their kids about Long Covid—and they have failed.

With Covid-19 circulating freely and repeatedly throughout the world, everyone needs to know that Long Covid can come from just one "mild" case of Covid, that there is no effective treatment, some of the very serious disabling conditions it causes are known to be lifelong, and that it's not as rare as most people believe. Long Covid is why the American Medical Association calls each Covid infection "akin to playing Russian roulette."[11]

> *"LC takes time to rear its ugly head. It is not like after the acute phase a switch flips and you have LC. You can see a clear progression over time and it becomes the most prevalent after 9 months. I have known many sufferers since early in the pandemic and it still surprises them*

with new symptoms and more frequent manifestations." —Joseph Eastman, Pathogen Update: 9-5-2024

Logically, every single person who has had Covid should be warned to look for the signs of Long Covid. The onset of Long Covid usually shows up in one of two ways. One is where someone has a Covid infection where symptoms never go away completely; this is considered Long Covid at around four weeks. The other is when someone experiences a Covid infection and then feels recovered, with Long Covid symptoms beginning at around four or as late as 12 weeks.

Here are some additional things we wish everyone knew about Long Covid:

• There is no "typical" person with Long Covid.
• Long Covid is life-changing and incurable (at this point in time).
• We don't know what Long Covid looks like after five years.
• We don't know what Long Covid will do to children as they grow up.
• Long Covid doesn't care how "healthy" you are.
• It's not anyone's fault for having Long Covid.
• People with Long Covid are not making it up.
• Some with Long Covid live with awful and ongoing internal and muscular pain, and may experience light, sound, smell, taste, and texture sensitivity as pain.
• Long Covid can give people gastrointestinal problems that may make them feel ashamed or embarrassed.
• Long Covid "fatigue" is more like getting hit by a truck than just "feeling tired."
• Expending energy for someone with Long Covid can come at considerable cost, sometimes setting back their recovery or causing them

to "crash" for days at a time, sometimes in a way so debilitating they can barely function.
• Exercise can cause harm and create health setbacks.
• Rates of Long Covid are double in disabled populations.
• "Brain fog" can make reading and writing (and screen time) difficult if not excruciating. It can cause someone to forget commitments, tasks, even conversations.
• People with Long Covid can't predict good or bad days.
• Those with Long Covid may be reluctant to tell you about it.
• People with Long Covid don't want to be asked if they've tried turmeric, yoga, reading a self-help book, or "manifesting."

The estimate of 400 million people reporting experiences with Long Covid worldwide (2024) is almost certainly an undercount. This due to lack of access to medical care, insurance denials, lack of acceptance about the disease, that people are not being made aware of the disease, stigma and bias in society about symptoms and the pressure to "feel fine" after an infection, systemic racism, ableism, misogyny, parents who were told kids don't get Long Covid, a glaring absence of medical competency around Long Covid, and medical gaslighting.

COVID AND MEDICAL GASLIGHTING

Medical gaslighting has been—and still is—the biggest barrier for getting help and healthcare for anyone and everyone experiencing Long Covid.[12] Medical gaslighting is when healthcare professionals invalidate, dismiss, or ignore concerns and symptoms. Often, the healthcare worker will attribute symptoms to a psychological or emotional condition.[13]

Medical gaslighting is important for partners and loved ones of people with Long Covid to understand so they better know what their loved one is going through. Your partner, or friend, or family member, needs to know that it's not "just you" nor is it possible for you to easily or safely get healthcare, let alone find doctors who acknowledge Long Covid, despite how common it has become. If you're reading this as the person with Long Covid, you may already be aware of most everything in this section, but may find it helpful to hand to someone to help them better understand what millions (if not hundreds of millions) of people just like you are dealing with.

Researchers at the Pacific Institute on Pathogens, Pandemics and Society published a research brief in 2023 showing that when Long Covid sufferers experienced gaslighting from medical practitioners, it extended "into community networks of family and friends who may also dismiss their symptoms, contributing to further stigmatization at home."[9] They added, "Medical gaslighting can present additional barriers to treatment, such as not being referred to specialists or Long Covid clinics. This can, in turn, compound other symptoms such as fatigue, and exacerbate the psychological symptoms of Long Covid, such as depression and anxiety."

The Conversation explained, 'Medical gaslighting can present additional barriers to treatment, such as not being referred to specialists or long COVID clinics. This can, in turn, compound other symptoms such as fatigue, and exacerbate the psychological symptoms of long COVID, such as depression and anxiety."[12] *The Conversation* added that gender biases play a strong role in preventing women from having their symptoms believed and poses a serious barrier to accessing care for Long Covid.

The facts bear this out. Especially BIPOC and disabled women are more likely to experience Long Covid medical gaslighting.[14] Patients are interrupted, blamed, humored, shamed, stigmatized, and denied medications; critical diagnosis are missed or done "too late" for treatments and interventions that would have worked. It is also deeply traumatizing. It leads to patients needing to plan extensively for their own safety before appointments or emergency trips, and don't feel safe going alone. Long Covid gaslighting is a significant, potentially deadly barrier to healthcare access.[15]

Compound that with deeply rooted, aggressive societal Covid denial and we've got the unnecessary suffering of hundreds of million of people, including children, worldwide. Covid medical gaslighting, and notably Long Covid medical gaslighting, is like medical—and racial—gaslighting on steroids. Long Covid's pervasive racist and ableist discrimination in particular has brought medical gaslighting to the forefront.[16] As *MIT Technology Review* described in 2022, "We've only just begun to examine the racial disparities of Long Covid."[17]

In the online publication *Long Covid: An Anthropological Perspective* medical anthropologist Emily Mendenhall comments on an interview with Black woman physician and leader in health justice Dr. Oni Blackstock, saying:

> "In this conversation Dr. Blackstock opened up a whole can of worms I've been trying to untangle: why is ME/CFS and Long Covid so commonly reported and amplified for white women (as well as men) while we have evidence that Black and Brown Americans are experiencing the same or worse symptoms? Blackstock explained that it's being a person or color and being a woman—'it's a double whammy of not getting care.'"[18]

Those with Long Covid also face ableism in medical gaslighting; disabled and chronically ill people know the phrase "but you don't look sick" all too well.[20] This is especially seen with Long Covid POTS and ME/CFS; these patients are commonly attacked, dismissed, and denied care by having their concerns and symptoms dismissed as "feelings."[19]

The movement to fight Long Covid gaslighting is global. So many were suffering from Long Covid and being gaslit that in mid-2020, "Long-haulers had to set up their own support groups," reported Ed Yong for *The Atlantic*.[21] "They had to start running their own research projects. They formed alliances with people who have similar illnesses, such as dysautonomia and myalgic encephalomyelitis, also known as chronic fatigue syndrome. A British group—LongCovidSOS—launched a campaign to push the government for recognition, research, and support."

Long Covid remains a struggle against medical and societal gaslighting, ableism and racism, as well as all efforts to thwart Covid-19 prevention.

EMOTIONAL AND COGNITIVE SYMPTOMS

The emotional and cognitive symptoms experienced by people with Long Covid are not as widely discussed as they should be, but a growing number of therapists and counselors worldwide are expanding this area. It's important for us to understand the impact of Long Covid's emotional and cognitive symptoms in order to know how it's affecting our relationships, whether you're the person with Long Covid, or the friend or loved one of someone with the condition.

Cognitive issues are common, as documented by the NIH in 2022 as: "Fatigue and cognitive dysfunction, such as concentration problems, short-term memory deficits, general memory loss, a specific decline in attention, language and praxis abilities, encoding and verbal fluency, impairment of executive functions, and psychomotor coordination, are amongst the most common."[22] Psychiatric issues can include depression, anxiety, trauma response, and PTSD. However, Long Covid fatigue should be renamed: the life-crashing experience is devastating for many and it is not "just" fatigue.[23]

Similarly, the "brain fog" that grips Long Covid sufferers is more than its name implies and can make everyday tasks as simple as grocery shopping or making a meal traumatically hard at times.[24] "Long-haulers with brain fog say that it's like none of the things that people—including many medical professionals—jeeringly compare it to," reported Ed Yong in *The Atlantic*. "It is more profound than the clouded thinking that accompanies hangovers, stress, or fatigue. For Davis, it has been distinct from and worse than her experience with ADHD. It is not psychosomatic, and involves real changes to the structure and chemistry of the brain. It is not a mood disorder."

Grief is a core component of the emotional interior of someone experiencing Long Covid. This can include feelings of loss about their health, career, sense of self-worth, independence, and more. Grief over loss of plans plays an enormous factor, too, like vacations that can't be taken or keep getting rescheduled, or larger life plans like career moves or family planning. Long Covid symptoms can cycle unpredictably and this can contribute to loss of social life, leading to feelings of grief over things like lunch with a friend that has to be canceled when symptoms flare.

Loss of relationships and intense feelings of grief can also come when friends and family are not as supportive—or disbelieve—the person coping with Long Covid. It's understandable that someone with Long Covid may not tell friends and family that they have it, simply because Long Covid is very confusing and difficult to explain. Going to events or meeting up with friends takes much more effort than it did before, and people with Long Covid often feel like they have to pretend to be their old selves in order to participate—only to feel completely drained or even set back afterward. It sometimes feels like it's just easier to stay home and decline to participate in having a social life.

Long Covid impacts ability, family, social life, and sense of self. It's very difficult to work or job hunt with an unexpected and widely misunderstood (for now) condition. Financial anxiety is a chief issue for many dealing with Long Covid, on top of finding and accessing healthcare providers who may not take you seriously (but will take your money).

Another significant anxiety stressor is the fact that someone with Long Covid must absolutely do everything possible to avoid a Covid reinfection and are forced to navigate a present-day where most people, including healthcare professionals, have views shaped by messaging that Covid concerns are "fringe" or trivial, that it's "just a cold," and all the unscientific fallacies that have cultivated a culture of resistance to Covid-19 prevention practices (and facts). There are many documented instances of Long Covid clinics and studies where participants have quit or avoided seeking care after discovering a lack of (or refusal) to do Covid-19 prevention basics, like masking.

Fighting to avoid reinfection becomes its own trauma and adds to Long Covid's psychological trauma response, which can also include PTSD around initial infection experiences, fear and trauma of diagnosis with Long Covid, and fear about the future.

It's all understandably isolating, and gives us clues about how alone someone with Long Covid can feel even in a supportive relationship, surrounded by caring family, or has understanding friends. You just feel stuck. Many are finding that connecting with others online in group support is a good way to get unstuck.

Some people might look at the words "groups" and recoil at the idea of talking about how you feel with strangers. I get it: being sick, gaslit, scared, feeling alone, and maybe helpless or even hopeless doesn't make me feel like "sharing my feelings" with anyone!

But consider this: the virtual Long Covid support groups run by Julia Centrella, Psy.D. at ChristianaCare are where people are connecting with people dealing with the same conditions and comparing self-care notes.[25] Noticing progress and small victories is hard and Long Covid messes with your sense of self; the groups mainly focus on improving quality of life. Common themes of discussion include symptoms, therapies, treatments, coping strategies, financial difficulties, social struggles, family impacts, not being taken seriously, and just having a place where they don't have to explain themselves or Long Covid.

Dr. Centrella advises that any group you consider should be run by someone familiar with Long Covid and up to date on the latest research and findings.

HOW LONG COVID CAN AFFECT RELATIONSHIPS

The impact of Long Covid on intimate partner relationships varies, ranging from adding strain to radically impacting and changing relationship dynamics. Living with chronic illness and disability can bring changes with relationship roles, expectations, plans, and the couple's relationship to the world—the identity of the couple.

For some, Long Covid might become like an unwanted third person in the relationship that the couple has to figure out how to live with, or live around. It's compounded by Long Covid's stigma, medical confusion and need to fight for acknowledgement and care, and uncertainty.

Most couples adjusting to Long Covid in the partnership had no idea any of this might happen to them, let alone how to suddenly become a caregiver, or how to fight for treatment against doctors who refuse to take Covid-19 or Long Covid patients seriously. Saying it can add "strain" in even the most solid, connected, supportive relationships is an understatement.

Long Covid can change everyday agreements couples have already made, such as who is able to do (or can remember to do) household chores. Long Covid will delay a couple's plans. Dates and appearances may need to change or must be canceled. How couples approach life with Long Covid requires extra planning, patience, flexibility, empathy, and communication that helps you check in with each other to avoid feelings of isolation, burden, resentment, or worse.

Stressors emerge when one partner has Long Covid and the couple might pivot and tackle the changes as a team, or not, or some uncertain combination of the two. One of the significant challenges people with Long Covid face is that they are disabled but people think they don't "look sick," or their cycling, coming-and-going-and-returning symptoms are interpreted as something that undermines the severity of their condition. People may feel like their partners don't believe them.

Disability and chronic illness, and especially Long Covid that can present inconsistently, is still being understood, and is the subject of minimizing and denial, can be fertile ground for intimate partner abuse. Partners may weaponize Long Covid to perpetuate controlling behaviors, compounding feelings of being unable to leave. Abuse specific to care relationships—like children and parents, or disabled people and paid attendants—is also a big problem here. Abusive behaviors may take the form of ignoring requests for masking and Covid-19 prevention practices, siding with minimizers, or deepening rifts around different levels of precaution.

Some relationships end. Some go on pause. Some pivot and continue in different forms, finding a closeness, unity, and intimacy centered on resiliency, communication, and caring.

Even in the most connected of relationships, Long Covid's physical and emotional effects cause sex lives to shift, get redefined, adapt, and evolve.

Unfortunately, I think it'll be a long time until we see open, accurate, and sex-positive discussion around Covid-19 and Long Covid's effects on sexual functioning and desire, both solo and within relationships. Like with many aspects of Covid's mass-disabling event, disabled people and disability activists have already done heaps of vital, inclusive work that can guide us where we might want to go. Or not go! Long Covid and sexuality is going to be something we learn about as we go along, and this includes figuring out what works and what doesn't.

In *The Ultimate Guide to Sex and Disability* by Miriam Kaufman, Fran Odette, and Cory Silverberg, the authors offer a comprehensive intimacy and pleasure primer for people with disabilities or chronic pain, illnesses or chronic conditions. The text is inclusive of age, gender, and orientation, aiming to help readers find what works for them across a range of disabilities found in Long Covid's symptom clusters, including ME/CFS.

Another great resource to consider when exploring Long Covid and sexuality, particularly regarding Long Covid's trauma and PTSD aspects, might be *Healing Sex: A Mind-Body Approach to Healing Sexual Trauma* by Staci Haines. Its focus is primarily on female childhood abuse survivors with an inclusive all-orientation approach, yet its body-based approach to healing is concretely helpful for anyone navigating dissociation, consent and boundaries, trauma triggers, and the emotions of healing. Partners of people with Long Covid may find it helpful, too.

I also highly recommend *Disability Intimacy: Essays on Love, Care, and Desire*, edited by Alice Wong. It's the follow-up to *Disability Visibility*, which also includes aspects of disability and intimacy that might shed some light on sexuality and Long Covid, be it in a relationship or single, and both books span genders, orientations, ages, abilities, and backgrounds. *Disability Intimacy* is packed with powerful, inspiring, and illuminating writing with a holistic approach to intimacy and connection, fantasies and realities, and centering sexuality when everything conspires to make us feel isolated and unconnected.

PARTNER ABUSE AND LONG COVID

Little attention has been paid to intimate partner abuse and Long Covid. Considering how clearly the demographics of Long Covid and intimate partner abuse overlap, disproportionately affecting women, BIPOC, and disabled—and how large (and growing) the populations are—it could very well be a crisis. Monash University (Australia) did one of the only studies on "the previously unseen impacts of Long Covid on individuals experiencing domestic violence" in January 2024, concluding that "each of these conditions worsened an individual's experience of the other."[26]

In the study, most had contracted Covid-19 in 2022; just over half were experiencing abuse in the relationship prior to their infection, and the rest "experienced abuse for the first time following their Long Covid diagnosis." Unlike the United States, which had a "pause" and shelter-in-place, Australia experienced strict lockdowns, which contributed to social isolation within the relationships—partner isolation is a hallmark of control for abusers. Most "participants believed contracting Long Covid had put them at higher risk of abuse due to a range of factors, including reduced brain functioning, low self-worth, social isolation associated with Covid restrictions, and the burden of care placed on their partners." The study, while still the only of its kind, shows that domestic violence services should have been a key component of pandemic prevention measures.

Instead, they were an afterthought. Some of us remember when much ado was made about addressing intimate partner abuse when we all stayed put to stop the spread and control the virus, but this, like controlling the virus, was a disastrously unfinished thought. "Victim-survivors described how their partners weaponised or manipulated their Long Covid symptoms to perpetrate abusive behaviours," wrote the Monash researchers. "Perpetrators exploited the mental and physical impacts of Long Covid to further entrap victim-survivors in coercively controlling relationships."

Those experiencing abuse told the researchers Long Covid had made them unable to leave their partner, and their symptoms made domestic abuse services inaccessible. "Addressing this issue requires workers responding to domestic violence to be alive to the complex intersection of chronic illness, ableism, and gender-based violence," Monash wrote.

COVID PERSONALITY CHANGES

> "After a few Covid infections, a year of no precautions, and no shortage of powerful propaganda, people I love are no longer recognizable. They've become entirely new people, and it's not just from 'moving on.' This is something else. These are dramatic personality changes."
> —Laura Miers (@LauraMiers, Oct 22, 2022)

WE'VE ALL HAD THAT one friend who was extremely careful and safe, knowing all the risks and dangers, then got Covid and suddenly decided it was no big deal and stopped masking. Or stopped caring about reinfection (or caring about infecting others). Some people have even forgotten how bad their initial infection really was—or how many times they've had Covid. Social media abounds with posts about this, some openly wondering whether a Covid infection has changed some people's personalities. This chapter recognizes these trends and lines of enquiry around people behaving differently (notably, in ways that don't align with their previous values) after having Covid and what's being said about understanding any changes.

It's baffling that some people go high-risk after getting Covid-19 a first, second, or even third infection. I'm not talking about people who believe "the government" is going to abduct them and give them "the jab," or mask burners, or any of the more socially accepted versions of anti-prevention dickishness. A 2022 study, "Personality and Individual Differences" looked at this population, concluding that "aspects of psychopathy and sadism were associated with less compliance with protective measures and more health/safety risk taking. Aspects of Machiavellianism were associated with less willingness to get vaccinated."[1]

None of that is particularly surprising. Though I think none of us expected to encounter a phenomenon where some of our empathetic, science-forward, Covid-conscious friends seem to stop being all of those things after the acute phase of a Covid-19 infection is over. Did the Covid change them? Were they hiding something from us? Are they trying to cut us out of their lives? Is it a kind of post-infection risk fatigue? Many of us are struggling to answer the question of "why" someone flips and starts engaging in (sometimes callously) high-risk behaviors, because it feels like we've lost a friend.

Most of my friends have had Covid. Many more than once. Most of my friends also have Long Covid now. In May 2023 I wrote: "I've only noticed a personality change in one friend. I haven't talked to him about it because we've grown apart since. He became uncharacteristically uncaring about masking and avoiding reinfection, and also about masking around others (like me). It's like his symptoms left with his empathy and impulse control." Over a year later, I can say that I've experienced marked behavioral changes in multiple friends struggling with Long Covid—observed and processed with their friends and loved ones—that align with research about Covid's post-acute-infection psychiatric symptoms, like delay discounting, a high-risk behavior in which immediate satisfaction is prioritized when making decisions.

However, it's important to understand that while some newly careless people are ending up with Covid's psychiatric baggage left behind, others aren't. There are a number of social conditions and inherent-human-nature things factoring into why someone previously Covid-cautious would flip after an infection and hop on the Reinfection Express (destination: Long Covid).

WHY DO SOME PEOPLE GIVE UP?

Obviously, people's perception of Covid-19's risks has changed over time. This is heavily influenced by misinformation coming from public health sources and media outlets pushing a vaccine-only prevention strategy, belief in a nonexistent "herd immunity," long Covid dismissal and denial, and normalization of high levels of infection and death. "Back to normal" messaging encourages aligning Covid with colds and flu, which fosters inaccurate public perceptions of Covid's harmlessness.

"I got it and I'm fine" is a dangerously subjective viewpoint with a virus that is proven to do temporary or lasting brain injury, but here we are. Someone might read ten articles on the grievous impact of Long Covid but then have one friend say "I heard it's not that big a deal anymore, all you do is take Paxlovid" –and what they take away is "Covid is no big deal." Where their minimizing friend "heard it's not a big a deal anymore" is where we can lay blame for that selection bias. We've been hammered–for years now–with Covid spin about "mildness" and "severity," and pre-messaged about new variants being "less severe" before data on severity had even been published. *The New York Times* claimed that the deadly Omicron wave was going to be "less severe" in 2021.[2] It's not hard to see that messing with public understanding of disease severity harmed people's ability to assess Covid risk before, and after, infections.

When someone is gaslit from every angle, "othered" and shut out from social interactions, and is being conditioned to doubt their judgment about health risks, gets Covid and wants very badly to "feel fine" like everyone says they should... it can change a few things. For one, an infection after vigilance can affirm feelings of helplessness and convince someone that mitigations are ineffective or pointless. The persuasive argument of "eventuality" with both infection and reinfection is certainly responsible for a lot of suffering, disability, and death.

Another reason someone might drop mitigations is simply because they got Covid and survived, or got off with an asymptomatic infection. This reaches back to the earlier trauma of first-year Covid-19. In comparison to 2020 it feels like a milestone. Like they "got away with it."

This can result in two risk-reduction outcomes. In one, the experience fuels an inherent optimism bias we all have hardwired into our weird little human heads, the belief that "it won't happen to *me*." Like when people dismiss the looming threat of Long Covid from reinfections "because I'm healthy" despite all evidence to the contrary, like the mounting number of Olympic athletes coping with the condition. Optimism bias is a huge problem in public health. Optimism bias is a huge problem in cybersecurity too, where people tasked with protecting systems always find themselves swimming upstream in a river of (always, eventually, mistaken) users who truly believe they'll never get hacked.

In another "I got it and it wasn't that bad" scenario, it can cause someone to change their overall risk assessment of Covid-19 and re-shape their attitude about risk reduction activities.

On their blog *Essays you didn't want to read*, JTO Ph.D. wrote:

> "Even when people do see suffering and death of others, personal experience can be more relevant and persuasive in the formation of beliefs and attitudes about risk reduction. I recently spoke with a nurse who has cared for Covid patients in the ICU. She has seen some Bad Stuff. But when she herself got Covid, she was asymptomatic, and that experience has disproportionately influenced her belief that vaccines aren't necessary, because the virus is 'so mild.'"[3]

JTO asked the question we all have: why on Earth would anyone who knows better risk reinfection? "But what about all the people who presumably *knew* that mask wearing and other forms of Covid risk mitigation were important for them personally (because, after all, they were doing it), yet suddenly stopped once they'd had an encounter with the virus? Wouldn't that *personal experience* make them even more committed to avoiding another infection?"[4]

The answer lies in our tendency toward binary thinking, like when people say they won't mask *at all* because they "can't mask forever" or that any Covid-19 mitigations in society whatsoever are equal to lockdowns. "To some unknown degree," wrote JTO, "people may be dropping their masks after recovery from infection with SARS-CoV-2 simply because the thing they were trying to accomplish ('never getting Covid') is now off the table, and in that all-or-nothing way of thinking in which people are so often inclined to engage, they feel they're no longer playing the *same game*—so they don't feel the need to play at all. This pattern of response contributes to recidivism within a whole host of health risk reduction realms, from weight management to the abstinence from alcohol and illicit drugs. (Unfortunately, messages from the Covid cautious community that people must engage in consistent risk avoidance *all the time*, without allowing for relapse, don't help this situation.)"

POST-COVID COGNITIVE CHANGES

There are other theories as to why our previously Covid-averse friends stopped caring about getting Long Covid, or who they infect, after an infection. Following a Covid infection, people may be more likely to engage in risky behavior because of psychological and/or neurological effects of the virus itself. "While basic personality tends to remain constant throughout adult life, conditions that disrupt brain function can induce extreme shifts in personality—and evidence is mounting that this happens for some people who contract Covid-19," reported *National Geographic* in 2022.[5]

A Covid infection, as well as Long Covid, are known to cause a range of cognitive and neuropsychological problems of varying severity and duration in some, but not all, people. "It doesn't help," reported *Rolling Stone* in 2021 on the bouts of sudden rage people might experience, "that 'personality change' means different things to different people—ranging from a dramatic transformation, to someone getting angry and frustrated more than usual."[6]

"Brain fog" can play a role here, too—though it's important to remember that Covid's "brain fog" is *not caused* by a mood or psychological disorder.[7] Considered common after a Covid-19 infection, "brain fog" symptoms are known to include poor memory, impaired concentration, difficulty thinking, impaired speed of information processing, and affects problem-solving abilities. What's important to understand is how "brain fog" makes people feel: it is a struggle, they feel they have to hide it, and doing basic things, like Covid prevention routines, are both incredibly hard and cost a lot of energy.

A wealth of research about Covid-19's cognitive effects began emerging in mid-2023 firmly establishing Covid infection—of any severity—as likely to leave lasting cognitive effects behind, including deficits in attention, executive function, memory, and learning, as well as sleep disorder.[8] "We now know that SARS-CoV-2 can damage any part of the brain," said a 2024 report in *Infection Control Today*.[9] "COVID-19 patients also demonstrate behavioral and executive dysfunction. The latter term means patients have difficulty in critical thinking, such as compromising and reaching a consensus, and difficulties in controlling antisocial behavior and determining when to become aggressive."

As with most things Covid, people who are more vaccinated and boosted, and didn't end up hospitalized with Covid, have less incidence of facing potential cognitive deficits and accompanying behavioral changes.[10]

Per *Sleep and Breathing Physiology and Disorders* (2023), Covid's cognitive impairment might stick around, but larger behavioral changes faded over a relatively short period.[11] "In a registry study of 236,379 Covid-19 survivors, about one-third of them received a neuropsychiatric diagnosis (such as stroke, dementia, insomnia, anxiety, and emotional disorders) within 6 months of the first symptoms of Covid-19, which is 44% higher than reported for influenza survivors." A 2022 study reported in *CellPress: Neuron* noted that, "In contrast to risk of cognitive impairment, the risk of anxiety and mood disorders normalized within 2 months following SARS-CoV-2 infection."[12] This might shed a little light on why some of our friends stop caring after an infection, but later decide that they do, in fact, want to care about being Covid-conscious again. It's another good reason to welcome back people who dropped masking and decide to pick it back up again.

Mood disorders and personality changes stemming from Covid-19 infection or Long Covid remain among the least discussed, especially with an understanding of how we might encounter and cope with them in daily life. For instance, a large 2024 study of Long Covid in South Korea and Japan showed a pronounced increase of Guillain-Barré syndrome, cognitive deficit, insomnia, anxiety disorder, encephalitis, ischemic stroke and mood disorder.[13]

Being mindful of Long Covid's tendency to increase anxiety and mood swings and how these might manifest can help us spot behavioral changes, keep an eye on friends who may need our support, and to counter and retrain any suspected changes. Perhaps in ourselves, too.

We might also find answers as to why we lost a prevention buddy to the "vax and relax" mindset by taking a closer look at one specific aspect of Covid's documented effects on the brain: delay discounting. In a 2022 study funded by the the Canadian Institutes of Health Research that examined Covid-19's links to cognitive function and psychiatric symptoms, researchers found:

"The results indicated that symptomatic Covid-19 was associated with the lower performance of cognitive tasks involving decision-making and executive function, with low scores in delay discounting and Flanker test scores, respectively... Delay discounting was also amplified in individuals with a history of symptomatic Covid-19. Delay discounting tasks are associated with the orbitofrontal cortex. These findings are significant as this region of the brain is thought to be the primary neuroinvasion and neuroinflammation site of SARS -CoV-2."[14]

That part about *amplified* delay discounting is crucial. Delay discounting is the inability to delay gratification, a consuming need for an immediate reward (or consequence) over a greater reward (or consequence) you'd need to wait for. Similar to diminished impulse control, if you say: "You can have $50 now or if you wait until tomorrow you can have $100," someone with amplified delay discounting will aggressively be unable to choose waiting for the better reward that comes a little bit later.

Delay discounting is a key element in understanding addiction, impulsive behaviors (the clinical kind), high-risk health decisions (think condoms and HIV), and ADHD. Per the American Psychological Association's *PsychNet*, "One of the most important areas in which discounting plays an important role is related to health."[15] It's interesting to note that the second study in that paper was a 2-wave population-wide survey where "baseline symptomatic Covid-19 history was associated with self-reported cognitive dysfunction and a latent variable reflecting psychiatric symptoms of anxiety, depression and agitation at [a 6-month] follow-up."

Amplified delay discounting in a Covid-19 context might look like someone who decides they no longer see the point in avoiding infection—and don't care about spreading Covid around, simply because they see no immediate benefits. They might also skip booster shots, because vaccination is in itself a type of investment in longer-term outcomes. Amplified delay discounting would absolutely play into the "Covid-YOLO" mindset, despite the alarming evidence piling up about Covid and reinfections, and long-term harms.

It could also explain why someone would go from being appalled by the US CDC's public health failures to then go out among people while still positive on a second or third infection, and when called on it, say something like "But the CDC says..." to excuse their (knowingly) harmful in-the-moment behaviors.

Post-infection amplified delay discounting and Covid's mood and anxiety symptoms after the acute infection are almost certainly playing out across many levels in wider society—especially with millions infected daily, nonstop, for months at a time, 2-3 times a year. I'm not trying to be a doomer here, I'm just saying that more people might be acting out and not realizing it, or knowing why.

Taken further, a 2022 piece in *Infection Control Today* explored the theory of a "Covid-19 Personality Disorder" and even theorized a link between Covid's behavioral changes and increasing social violence.[16] Noting a "marked increase in violent crimes in the United States and Canada, along with the plethora of mass killings and school shootings during the pandemic" the report said that in addition to the pandemic itself, "We must consider the possibility that the observed behavior aberrations may directly result from the infection and the central nervous system damage it has caused."

The 2022 article based its focus around Covid's cognitive effects and traffic accidents. Interestingly, Covid and car crashes was revisited in a 2024 *Neurology* study,[17] which found "an association between acute Covid-19 rates and increased car crashes" due to Covid's neurologic changes, cautioning neurologists to potentially consider post-acute Covid patients as "medically impaired drivers."

Setting aside the *Infection Control Today* article's annoying "during the pandemic" phrasing—hey buddy, we're sitting right here, still in it, thanks—the paper explained:

"This theory centers around damage to the frontal lobe in the area of the prefrontal cortex. A variety of emotional-social disturbances can occur with lesions to this area... 'Irritability, impatience, and lability are common manifestations along with deficits in abilities critical to interpersonal sensitivity and socially appropriate behavior, including deficient self-monitoring of social behavior' along with impairment with 'moral reasoning and judgment.' Dysexecutive personality disturbance can also occur which is associated with 'impaired cognitive control and the latter associated with deficits in emotional/social behavior and decision-making.'"

"In other words," they added, "the prefrontal cortex is involved in determining when aggression is and is not appropriate." I think the *Infection Control Today* article's answer to its own 'what can we do about it' question is correct but falls short—its advice is to avoid reinfection at all costs. Yep, got it, we're all #doingmybest out here.

So, what if you're worried about yourself or someone you care about? While I'm the first to point out that we don't know—yet—what Covid-19 does to the body after 5 years, it looks like (so far) the kinds of behavioral changes we're talking about here can recede over time. A late 2021 investigative piece in *National Geographic* interviewed one subject who had post-infection "impulsive" and "irrational behavior," and then developed paranoia. "For some patients, this so-called Covid psychosis resolves with time," *National Geographic* explained. Around six months later, "he'd fully recovered."

That's great, but you can't exactly tell someone wondering if Covid-19 gave them the parting gift of impaired impulse control to just "wait it out." It may provide some comfort around coping with friends who quit making and taking precautions. It's all the more reason for us to withhold judgment, and to be chill prevention besties when they start masking again.

If you're wondering whether or not you might be affected, what we can do now is figure out how to self-assess, make a plan to deal with in-the-moment stuff, and if we think it's really happening to us, we can use tools to re-train our brains and speed up the recovery process.

First: Self-assess—or talk to a trusted friend or therapist about how you've been reacting to life since your initial infection. Try to think of a recent situation where you chose between long or short-term gain. Set aside shame for a moment and consider any recent situation where you may have "snapped" or lashed out at someone. Are you more easily overwhelmed than before? Have you taken risks you wouldn't have before, or done things you worried about afterward? Have your decisions or behaviors put anyone else at risk? To all of these queries, ask yourself why.

It's hard to catch yourself, but when you're making decisions or embarking on a risk, try asking yourself why you need to. ADHD impulse control tips and techniques can help. *Psych Central* and *Positive Psychology* have terrific tools to check yourself before you wreck yourself (or someone else) in the moment, including practicing how to recognize when you're about to behave in a way where it's actually the leftover Covid-19 driving, and not you. Covid can't drive. Get out of the car, Covid.

Look in the "References and Resources" chapter for additional tools.

Not everyone is "into" therapy or counseling, but if you're concerned or even just wondering about having any post-infection cognitive detritus hanging around, it's always better to talk to a professional. Your friends and loved ones are important as your support team. But they're not trained to handle counseling conversations or help you sort mental stuff out, and they're also dealing with their own stuff.

It's clear that Covid-19 is causing personality changes for some people, seen both in the mounting evidence and our lived experiences. The disease itself does it, but I think we shouldn't discount the trauma of the sickness itself. That includes the mental and emotional toll of the pandemic and its oft-devastating gaslighting, the loneliness of being the only people masking or just trying not to get Covid, the insurmountable loss and grief of the past few years, and all the things we should be talking about and starting to process, but no one will talk about it. All of this, plus the complete abandonment by public health leadership—once again, we're out here with no map.

ISOLATION AND CONNECTION

> *"The silver lining in this literal dumpster fire of a pandemic is connecting with the most real, empathetic women I've had the privilege to encounter in my lifetime. Our bonds have been forged through survival & sacrifice to keep our families safe." —California Codes*

YOU CAN CATCH IT on a plane, you can catch it on a train. You can get it in a bar, you can get it in a car. You can catch it in a gym and if you go brunching on a whim. You can get it from a teacher, boss, or nurse, but from a friend it might hurt worse. Restaurant, party, conference, no matter; Covid just loves it when we gather.

One of the most insidious things about Covid-19 is that it spreads through social contact. The air we breathe isn't the only thing that sustains us; so is staying connected to other people. That's why everyone avoiding infection for the past five years has been thrust into an unprecedented prolonged limbo of social isolation. Lockdowns, shelter-in-place, and social distancing, were all prevention measures to stop social spread. But we needed to stabilize ourselves through connection: remote work and school, zoom socials, Facebook events, social media, Netflix watch parties, and gaming rushed in to fill our needs. In hacking and information security, these were essentially a "hotfix"—a quick, temporary update hurried out to fix a problem.

Little did we know that anyone avoiding infection would be stuck in varying states of social isolation for a very long time, with every Covid-cautious person wondering exactly how long Covid-Chella would have to go on until someone, anyone would tap the brakes on repeated mass infection.

Looking back at 2020, all of the self-help articles about coping with social isolation and loneliness, and how both would need to be addressed for post-pandemic societal mental wellness, now seem quaint.

Those articles seem quaint in a cynical way now because those of us currently in some form of preventative social isolation remember how connected we felt when *everyone* wanted to prevent infection. We had to keep apart but we were doing it together, to keep ourselves and each other safe. There was a feeling of belonging in seeing that all the people in your neighborhood cared for each other. In Aotearoa New Zealand, it was a "team of five million" in lockdowns and an overall feeling of people working together toward a common good and a shared future. We felt this in parts of the US, too.

It was up to leadership and public health officials to keep this going and push back against the forces that wanted to spread Covid and divide us. But when leadership pivoted to an ineffective vaccine-only strategy, removed all protections, and encouraged opposition to prevention while the disease mutated, disabled, continued killing—our unity was shattered. "I miss the feeling that people cared about us medically vulnerable people," posted SG. "Now we are living like ghosts."

In our era of zero Covid protections and hostile mockery toward prevention, social isolation is essentially being forced on people who don't want to get infected. "Do I not deserve to live a life that is free from the constant threat of reinfection with a virus that already took so much from me?" Julia Doubleday wrote for *The Gauntlet*.[1] "Do I have the right to socialize, to eat in a restaurant? After all, isn't that what the people who refuse to mask claim? That a life without eating indoors is a life that isn't worth living? What about the millions of people who were disabled by their first, second or third Covid infections? Do they deserve to risk reinfection each time they leave home?"

The burden of social isolation in order to avoid a Covid infection is heavy. Much like our disenfranchised Covid-19 grief, the social isolation we're enduring is going dismissed by most people in our lives, in addition to being considered socially unacceptable. Disabled people and those with chronic illness before the time of Covid have been coping with this hurtful BS and cultivating resilience around it pretty much since the dawn of time.

Before Covid-19, social isolation was viewed through some pretty narrow lenses. To generalize, it's more often described as a condition, rather than a situation. Articles about social isolation tended to focus on risks and treatment, rather than coping skills. And while society is primarily the perpetrator when it comes to social isolation and disabled people, social isolation in this context has been sidelined as a 'disabled problem.'

There were a few glimmers of hope about the inclusion of disabled people and chronically ill into new social isolation conversations people were having at the beginning of the pandemic. March 2020 saw *Forbes* publish "Disabled People Have Unique Perspectives On Solitude" by Andrew Pulrang, noting that this road was already well-traveled by disabled and chronically ill people.[2]

"Some say disabled people have valuable lessons to teach non-disabled people about going it on their own," Pulrang wrote. "Disabled people themselves agree, sometimes with a dose of bitter irony. But many of us are also worried we will be *left* on our own, without the help we need to meet our most basic needs." Fast forward to 2024 and that's exactly what happened. With the addition of tens—and globally, hundreds—of millions of people newly disabled by Long Covid, and untold further numbers remaining in social isolation to prevent infection. "Understanding the different ways disabled people process solitude has never been quite this relevant before," concluded Pulrang in what now reads like a prescient message in a bottle from the March that never ended for so many.

It wasn't really until two years into the pandemic that social isolation finally started to get a hotfix, however small. *Healthline* wrote in 2022, "Social isolation, in a nutshell, means your social network is limited and unfulfilling."[3] Well, that's closer! I'd call having to choose between Christmas with the family and potentially becoming bed-bound from Long Covid or getting new-onset diabetes a *bit* more than "unfulfilling," but sure. "Anyone can become isolated," they add. "To put it another way, isolation often has nothing to do with your character, charisma, or other personality traits."

Healthline goes on to describe other prolonged circumstances where people find themselves socially isolated, noting that our Covid-19 hotfixes (like remote work) have made it common for people to spend "entire days in solitude." Interestingly, the American Psychological Association noted in 2022 that: "[lockdowns, physical distancing and the switch to remote work and school] undoubtedly increased social isolation, but research has found that social isolation does not always lead to loneliness. Social isolation means having a small social network and few interactions with others, while loneliness is the painful feeling of having less or poorer quality social connections than a person wants."[4]

Social isolation is the situation we're in; loneliness is one of the ways it might make us feel inside. As the ongoing pandemic steamrolled ahead over lives and loves, Western countries pretty much tossed everyone who didn't want to get infected into a self-defense social isolation black hole after the vaccine rollout in May 2021, and haven't looked back since.

Other countries, each with their own pandemic denial problems, still realize they've got a problem on their hands when massive swaths of the population can't safely participate in society. The Japanese government established the "Public-Private Collaboration Platform for Tackling Loneliness and Isolation" in 2022, positioning social isolation as an urgent issue at the national level in the country's Covid-19 responses.[5] The end result is mainly a website for help and referrals, although it does acknowledge "issues related to loneliness and isolation have become increasingly evident as the Covid-19 pandemic continues" and "is truly a contemporary social problem that needs to be faced head-on."

THE OTHERING OF COVID PREVENTION

Not everyone will feel loneliness in social isolation of course, just as we know what it's like to feel lonely in a group of people. Similarly, the kind of social isolation we're experiencing by avoiding high-risk Covid settings isn't fixed on staying home all the time. The "othering" of people who take Covid precautions in public spaces is very much a thing many of us encounter that makes us feel even more isolated.

If you're unfamiliar with the concept of "othering", the Canadian Museum for Human Rights describes it as: "When we highlight differences between groups of people to increase suspicion of them, to insult them or to exclude them, we are going down a path known as 'othering'... Othering sets the stage for discrimination or persecution by reducing empathy and preventing genuine dialogue. Taken to an extreme, othering can result in one group of people denying that another group is even human."[6] Othering is a tool for social control used by those emboldened to split society into who is considered "normal" and who isn't.

Covid-cautious readers will find that this concept resonates with the social exclusion, gaslighting, and attacks faced upon encountering anti-maskers, glares and stares, or even being put at risk by friends and loved ones. Disabled people, chronically ill people, people of color, and queer folx already know: this is the street they live on.

Othering in a Covid-19 prevention context might look like:

- A barista ignoring a masked person for the customer behind them.
- Glaring, staring, or pointing.
- Refusing service or entry to a masked person.
- Treating a masked person with fear or distrust.
- Reluctance to interact with people taking precautions.
- Only allowing masks at events for medical conditions.
- Getting "the silent treatment" from frontline workers, like cashiers.
- Suggesting someone masked behave differently than others, such as wait outside.
- "Forgetting" to share information with (only) you.
- Excluding Covid-cautious people (or their kids) from invites.

- Event policies that "tolerate" masks ("masks are allowed if").
- Exaggerated gestures to "help you" understand.
- Past-tense pandemic phrasing when you're masking.
- Being excluded from conversation or polite idle chatter.
- Drawing negative attention to your mask.

"We also see 'othering' manifest as what appears to be passive, systemic indifference," wrote Kim Samuel, author of *On Belonging: Finding Connection in an Age of Isolation*. "This includes subtle cues of not belonging, like microaggressions of language and refusals to listen."

Othering is all about the comfort of the person doing the othering. For pandemic purposes, it's about playing "back to normal" against the person taking precautions in order to isolate them further. We could explore why someone might do it (ignorance, fear, pathological insecurity, Darwin Award-seeking, garbage fire bigotry, conspiracy theory brain worms), but what's more useful is recognizing that othering attempts to increase our feeling of Covid social isolation and cuts us off from our sense of pandemic resilience.

To flip the switch on what othering does to us, Samuel explains that we have to cultivate belonging. "To overcome othering and build shared belonging, we need to engage in work to realize a shared vision. When we have purpose—especially shared purpose—we're less subject to the feelings of 'estrangement' that Toni Morrison described."

THE NEW TOGETHERNESS OF PREVENTION

Don't get me wrong: I'm the last person who thinks we should all join hands and "Kumbaya" our way through this mess. I mean, if it helps, do it. I do agree with Kim Samuel on defying the harms social isolation and othering can do to our pandemic resilience by cultivating belonging. Because the reality is that staying Covid safe is a solo, lonely, and isolating way to move through the world right now, even if you have supportive friends and family. There's a huge, concerted effort at play to make us feel like we're the "only ones" who care about Covid-19, who still mask, that we're outsiders looking in on a world where life goes on without us. That we're alone. But nothing could be further from the truth—and that's easy to prove.

Finding community in the face of systemic Covid-19 denialism and the safety requirements of social isolation is the ultimate way to build pandemic resilience. Without community in a time of high risk and stress, we can feel distanced, depressed, disconnected, or even ill. You don't need to join a group if that's not your style. Simply taking stock of what people are doing around the world right now to push back anti-prevention forces might be enough to get you re-centered.

Take mask blocs for example: these are grassroots, community-led indie groups that distribute free high-quality masks, Covid-19 tests and other equipment for local communities. As of this writing, there are over 140 mask blocs worldwide—and the phenomenon is only around two years old. Those include Inverness (Scotland), Palm Beach (Florida), Wellington (Aotearoa), Lyon (France), Anchorage (Alaska), Montreal (Canada), Melbourne (Naarm; Australia), Sunset/San Francisco (California), Mask Bloc Éire (Ireland), Santiago (Chile), Hobart (Tasmania), London (England), and so many more.[7]

In addition to mask blocs, there are almost 90 indie Covid-19 prevention groups worldwide working toward education, awareness, clean air initiatives, and more. Like the rapid proliferation and success of mask blocs, it's proof that we can connect and stay safe, while showing the world a lot of people are not the "only ones" who care about Covid harms and prevention. Examples include Clean Air in

BC Schools (Canada), Dansk Covidforening (Denmark), Aotearoa Covid Action (New Zealand), AVICO Brasil, COVID Advocacy NY, Suomen Covid (Finland), Covid Action Australia, COVID Persistente Argentina, Long Covid Italia, COVID Safe Maryland, AMACOP (Spain), Millions Missing France, Long Covid Switzerland, and more in Netherlands, Canary Islands, Mexico, Belgium, Chile and... you get the (global) picture.

That list doesn't even include clean air orgs and virtual groups. There are a lot of databases out there: one way to start could be to search "still Coviding" along with your city, region, state, or country on the Covid Meetups website (meetup.com).[8] Look around online and locally, check the "References and Resources" chapter of this book (especially the global Covid Action Map), and you'll find more closer to home.[9] While Reddit can be terrible in various subreddits, the subs "Zero Covid Community", "Covid Grief", and "Covid-19 Support" are full of supportive posters and with people reaching out for connections (and accurate advice).

So as you can see, if you do find connecting with a group appealing there are several to choose from and many ways to participate, so you can take it at your own speed. Want to lurk and just feel less alone without interacting? Do you want to see how others are solving prevention problems or are fighting to get masks back in healthcare? You might microvolunteer or find ways to make your anger or sadness into productive energy by really getting involved. Your shared experience for a cause or shared interest means that you have things to share, and there will always be people dealing with the same problems you are.

Narrow your focus before you begin. Groups and communities fall into a few general categories and branch out into different goals: Clean air, masks, and Long Covid are examples that branch into mutual aid, activism, local focus on all aspects of prevention, healthcare activism, education, and information sharing. If you're not sure where to start, begin by seeing what's happening locally with mask blocs, clean air in schools groups, or Long Covid awareness. Even if schools aren't your thing, the community focusing on schools may know about other groups doing things you're more into.

Communities provide information and tools—and also keep your stress levels in check. Some will be a good fit for your time, energy, and emotional bandwidth, and some won't. Don't be afraid to shop around until you find something that "clicks" or changing groups if yours isn't working for you. Some groups may not be the right match for your location, ability, cultural background, or approach to a cause—and that's okay.

Being in a group can feel outsider-y or frustrating sometimes, and fighting back a pandemic can bring up difficult feelings. But remember: if you can help change just one mind about prevention, you've done one of the most significant acts to help turn this thing around.

MAKE ANGER USEFUL

"Whenever I hear the governments – and I use the term in plural deliberately – telling me I need to live with Covid, I'm filled with anger and frustration. I'm trying to, but you're not making it easy." —Dr. George Taleporos

WE ARE *STRUGGLING*. SELF-CARE proponents will tell us to meditate, "think positive," exercise more, do yoga, "get plenty of rest," and a myriad of other things which can be useful—but comes off as shallow and ineffective for a shared traumatic event that continues to unfold in real-time. Look, I'm the first person to turn off notifications, cuddle up with a large pizza and bottle of something, and binge comfort episodes of *Star Trek* after reading about the latest mask ban. It helps.

But before anyone slaps on a band-aid of "be nice to yourself" we first need to address how we're being affected.

We are living through a once-in-a-century, ongoing pandemic. Hundreds of millions are newly disabled. *The Economist* estimated as many as 30 million people worldwide died from Covid-19 in less than five years.[1] Social supports and prevention tools have been ripped away and many are convinced that "living with it" means that any number of us are disposable. This is a mass traumatic event. It affects us in ways consistent with other mass traumatic events, such as natural disasters and other disease outbreaks.

The American Psychological Association (APA) defines trauma as "any disturbing experience that results in significant fear, helplessness, dissociation, confusion, or other disruptive feelings intense enough to have a long-lasting negative effect on a person's attitudes, behavior, and other aspects of functioning. Traumatic events... often challenge an individual's view of the world as a just, safe, and predictable place."[2]

Here are some things you might feel:

- Anger
- Anxiety and fear
- Grief
- Overwhelm
- Detachment, as if you're an outsider to your own life
- Intense distress
- Unsafe, even when it makes no sense to feel this way
- Irritability
- Sadness
- Guilt, shame, and self-blame
- Mistrust and a sense of betrayal
- Depression and hopelessness

- Alienation, isolation and loneliness
- Embarrassment
- Helplessness

And here are some things you might experience:

- Roller coaster emotions
- Frustration or anger that disturbs your concentration
- Feeling "stuck" or trapped
- Feeling "watched" or harshly judged in public spaces
- Intrusive, upsetting thoughts or memories that can come on suddenly
- Unreliable memory, such as difficulty remembering exact details
- Nightmares, mask anxiety dreams, and insomnia
- Physical reactions such as a pounding heart, rapid breathing, nausea
- Difficulty concentrating
- Avoidance of people, events, or situations
- A "freeze" response, or overwhelm that feels paralyzing

It's okay to feel and experience all these things—they're normal reactions to what we're going through. You may only feel some of the things mentioned here, or you may feel all of them. Sometimes, just when you feel like you're doing okay, one trigger will bring back that feeling in your chest or your stomach, and the emotional spiral begins again. If you have a partner or loved one, make sure you show them this list so they know what you're feeling. Reading the list will give them an idea of what's going on when the internal storms come in and you get depressed, snap at them out of the blue, or toss and turn in bed.

You might feel like it will never end, but it will. It's tempting to give into the pro-infection mindset of binary thinking about our current circumstances, that this will go on like this "forever." Except that logic doesn't hold up under scrutiny. The waves of mass disability on stressed healthcare systems and looming cardiac crisis yoinking people out of workforces in every sector would like to have a word with leadership about entire populations having 2-3 Covid infections a year. And the truth is, time plus anything equals change.

Until then, here are some ways to deal with those feelings.

Many of us have been staying isolated or continue sheltering at home, and this robs us of our need to socialize, participate, feel like we belong, and feel connected. Talking to like-minded, Covid-safe people can help in magnitudes. That can happen in person with friends or at Covid-safe meetups, online in Covid-aware communities (like ones on Discord, Slack, Facebook, and more), or seek out Covid safety nerds on apps like Mastodon, Bluesky, Instagram, Threads, or other social media site. Talking to non judgemental people who care about you can help, as can talking to a counselor or therapist. Joining a support group may also comfort you and allow you to feel stronger about your decisions and space as you move through the world.

Self-isolating for long periods can contribute to "touch isolation" by reduced stimulation to a fundamental human sense. "I hope that by everyone experiencing some sort of touch isolation, the sense of touch will be shuffled to the forefront of our minds, in really believing it as a really important sense to help us navigate our environment and help us interact with one another," Neuroscientist Victoria Abraira told *CBC* in April 2020.[3]

Abraira recommended "paying more attention to things that feel good on the skin as a way to remedy touch isolation—especially for people who might find themselves home alone for extended periods of time." Physical self-care such as grooming, nail care, hair or makeup sessions, and skin care goes a long way to enhance your mental, emotional and physical wellbeing during long periods of isolation, as well as time with animal companions.

Doing things every day—especially small things—that make you feel good is important, as is finding a way to relax. Experiencing natural beauty will help ground you in the present and feel reconnected with places you love. Keeping a journal where you put your feelings into words also works for some people. Many people also find religious or spiritual practices help them cope. Try not to rely on drugs, alcohol, or caffeine, as these substances can make things worse.

If the way you feel just won't let up, and if it gets in the way of your important relationships, jeopardizes your job or schoolwork, or keeps you from functioning normally (especially if you feel like you just can't take it any longer), reach out to someone who is Covid-aware and will help you weather your storms until they're gone.

There is a growing international network of Covid-aware therapists, notably in the COVID-Conscious Therapist Directory (covidconscioustherapists.com); find someone to talk to who "matches" with you. That means finding someone who will also be culturally competent for you; therapy has an incredibly racist and ableist history and present so make a list of qualities you seek. Consult the *EEDA Newsletter Vol 5, Issue 5: How to Find a Therapist* for an excellent step-by-step guide: you'll find a link in the chapter "References and Resources."[4]

WHY WE FEEL ANGRY ABOUT COVID

Some of us are mad as hell about this situation—and for good reasons.

- Leadership has abandoned us to endless reinfection cycles.
- Public health has been regressed beyond a pre-pandemic level.

- We are denied access to data for disease surveillance.
- Some governments are making masking illegal.
- There is no support for Covid-specific prevention.
- Prevention and treatment are inaccessible and unaffordable for many.
- Covid guidance doesn't follow the science.
- Disabled and high risk people are sentenced to life in isolation and risk of death for basic services.
- Our elders are being pointlessly sacrificed.
- People are dying from catching Covid-19 in hospitals.
- The time where we cared as a society has been erased.
- Reporters are not vetting sources nor fact-checking data or claims.
- Covid minimizing and denial is eugenicist.
- BIPOC are disproportionately affected by Covid and multiple studies show white people take the least precautions.
- Lies about "endemic" "mild" and "herd immunity" are really obvious.
- Our trauma is from living through an ongoing pandemic, not from "lockdowns."
- People act like acknowledging Covid's risk is the problem.
- We're furious that leadership can't comprehend the effects of mass disability.
- Leadership and media are promoting revisionist history.
- Covid-19 is a preventable disease.
- Children's lives have been destroyed.

After looking over that list it's easy to see why anger is a pretty valid response. It would be odd if we *didn't* feel angry. Our voices calling for disease prevention and change have been characterized as pathologically angry, and we're constantly forced into situations where we have to swallow that anger to avoid infection, or beg leadership for Covid tools and prevention. People of color and disabled people bear the worst of it—two populations disproportionately impacted by the pandemic and Long Covid.

Psychiatrist Jonathan M. Metzl made a clear connection about this in *The Protest Psychosis*, his book documenting how Black Americans protesting for civil rights in the 1960s and 70s were diagnosed with (and medicated for) schizophrenia — the clinical definition hadn't changed, but instead equated Black anger with "mental illness."

Disabled and chronically ill people have long suffered the medicalization of their emotions, whose anger is also pathologized as an impairment effect, threat, or mental health disorder. In "Medicalizing disabled people's emotions—Symptom of a dis/ableist society" researcher Yvonne Wechuli explains: "Disabled people are, thus, instructed to change their feelings or even have them treated, rather than to criticize conditions that evoke anger in the first place."[5]

Yet we have every right to be angry. We didn't want to become mask fit-test specialists, we wanted to go back to doing things we loved. We didn't want to watch our friends become bed-bound in year three of the pandemic, we wanted to dance at their weddings.

What's important is what we do with it. That means taking a minute to acknowledge that yep, this makes me incredibly mad, again. Even just a moment of going "Grrrr I'm so angry" can be the difference in how you end up expressing that anger. Unacknowledged anger or feeling furious and pushing it down is how we end up inadvertently wasting time fighting with social media trolls, internalizing it into despair or depression, "freezing up" from overwhelm, and other counter-productive responses.

The point here is to decide if you want to do anything about this intense feeling in the moment, or cool off and do something about it later, or switch tracks entirely. "Fear warns us about danger, grief tells us to seek support, joy tells us that we should continue doing whatever it is that makes us feel good," wrote psychologist Jade Wu for *Psychology Today*. "Anger is the same. It tells us that injustice is being enacted, or that we need to take action to ensure the survival of our body and our integrity. People can steal, assault, cheat, bully, and oppress without an ounce of anger. But without anger, the victims would shrug and continue to endure injustice."[6]

COVID, MOURNING, AND GRIEF

Mourning is the external expression of loss, while grief is our internal experience of loss. We've been denied the time and space for both. Mourning was denied at first by the physical conditions of the pandemic itself, then by politicization. "The pandemic has replaced community with isolation, empathy with judgment, and opportunities for healing with relentless triggers," wrote Ed Yong in *The Atlantic*.[7] "It has opened up private grief to public scrutiny, all while depriving grievers of the collective support they need to recover… By upending the entire world, Covid could have created a shared experience that countered the loneliness of grief."

And for a moment it did. But we lost that, too.

Some of us have lost loved ones, whether from death, new disability, risk assessment, or emotional estrangement. Many have lost jobs, businesses, careers, livelihoods, and savings. Some have lost their homes. Many Covid-aware people have lost social and family connections, the necessary sustenance of socializing and participating in society and social rituals, and grieve the loss of inclusion, as well as our agency. Many now grieve the loss of their health and physical ability from one or multiple reinfections.

Anyone avoiding infection feels profound loss over having a baseline of safety in public spaces, or any trust once placed in healthcare or leadership. Social, racial, and physical inequities oppose our need to make tangible the scale of loss, and the social and emotional weight, of our multilayered grief.

It would help if we could mourn our losses. "After death, routine and social connection can help mourners cope," Yong wrote. "But grievers have been deprived of both because of America's continued failure to control the pandemic."

There is little recognition in any country of the profound grief people experienced and continue to experience around Covid-19. There are no official monuments to honor the dead and political divisiveness has denied loss by shifting blame onto those "at risk" and the deceased. We are unable to mourn when we can't gather safely in person. We are left to struggle for recognition of our losses. Mourners have been left to construct their own memorials, from The National Covid Memorial Wall in London[8] to online memorials, like Marked by Covid,[9] and the grassroots COVID-19 Monument Committee in Chicago.[10] Many of these efforts have been impeded or dismissed.

In 1989, Dr. Kenneth J. Doka first introduced the concept of disenfranchised grief as the process in which the loss is "not, or cannot be, openly acknowledged, publicly mourned, or socially supported."[11] It is when someone is "isolated in bereavement" and whose grief is not acknowledged by society. Bereavements that are not socially acceptable, stigmatized grief. Sound familiar?

In an excellent *Health Central* article, science writer Ilene Raymond Rush explains how disenfranchised grief isn't limited to death.[12] It applies to other losses we experience, including:

- Unacknowledged relationships

- Unrecognized loss, such as a divorce or coworker death

- When the grieving person is discounted (ageism, ableism, racism)

- Loss carrying stigma or embarrassment

- When the grief process doesn't fit with societal norms

Unfortunately, most advice on processing disenfranchised grief centers on the exit kinds of in-person interactions many of us are grieving and remain unable to access due to the loss itself, as well as health and safety risks.

Aside from that, *PsychCentral*'s "All About Disenfranchised Grief" has suggestions we can better adapt to our pandemic times.[13] Begin with "Know your loss is valid." You do not have to explain yourself to anyone, and you are the only one who gets to decide if your grief is valid. *PsychCentral* adds, "All thoughts and feelings you have about a loss are valid regardless of whether they're expressed or received as valid by others." Let yourself grieve: give yourself all the time and space you need to process the loss.

Memorialize your loss. Make a photo album (private or for sharing), or an online tribute post, even if it's not specific. Consider creating a ritual. We may not be able to visit that restaurant we once shared with a friend we miss, but we can ritually recreate the meals we shared at home. Visit a Covid-safe location that has meaning, watch a film or listen to a song that marks your grief, leave a token, like flowers, at an important spot. Some mark their grief with rituals of community care, like mask and test distribution or "thank you for masking" handouts.

Next, seek support. Try to connect with others experiencing something similar, such as online Long Covid support groups,

Covid-19 memorial organizations, or even anonymous forums like r/COVIDgrief ("Welcome to the club you hate being a part of") or r/COVID19_support. Check the "Resources chapter for more. Find ways to release your feelings, like in writing. *PsychCentral* suggests finding a therapist — I'll add that shopping for a Covid-conscious therapist is critical here.

INFORMATION OVERWHELM

Staying safe in a literal pandemic would be easier if we didn't feel overwhelmed by Covid-19 disinformation, ignored surges, disappearing data, mask bans, report after report about Covid's harms, and constant news of public health leadership making yet another disastrous decision not to prevent the spread of the virus.

We can stand by our boundaries, be fierce allies, educate for awareness, work toward change in public health, fight Covid injustice, hand out masks, and all the things we see ourselves doing to turn this thing around when we feel hopeful and strong. But a lot of us are reeling from the violence of our abandonment to a terrible, frightening disease the world still has yet to fully understand. Meanwhile, news and social media algorithms specialize in surfacing the most upsetting things when we least need it. A lot of people feel scared, angry, and depressed, worriedly checking news and social media for the next bit of bad news.

We shouldn't check out or look away. Staying informed is critical for our survival, especially when part of our survival means sharing information about even the most basic things, like where to find N95 masks.

Yet we also have to stay present and grounded, which means balancing our information intake with our mental and emotional well-being.

Begin by narrowing your interests to specific topics. Are masks your thing? That's where you can go deep. Is air quality confusing? That's okay—it doesn't need to be your mission. Examples include surge tracking, mask bans, Long Covid, vaccine equity, masks in healthcare, Covid and workplace safety, disability justice, clean air in schools, mask blocs, or other aspects of the pandemic you resonate with. This way, you can narrow your focus and set aside the urge to take everything in, the urge to feel responsible to do something about everything. For instance, you might choose to stay up to date on the latest studies on masking while relying on a trusted friend, colleague, acquaintance, or trusted Covid news source for the latest info on clean air or booster shot developments.

Clean house. Remove information sources that make your feeds repetitive, and ones that are more sensationalism than informed reporting. You may also want to remove sources that make you feel pissed off or upset, such as ones that minimize or downplay Covid-19, oppose prevention tools, use "post-pandemic" language, or push Covid gaslighting.

Ask yourself: is this source actually helping inform me? If so: what are they informing you about, exactly? Do they use all-caps, use the word "BREAKING" without providing a citation, resurface old information for clicks, or court outrage? Dump them or move them to a list you can optionally check so they're not in your face. Consider following individual people (like reporters, organizations, or activists whose prevention levels are the same as yours) that share news as it happens. Follow people who help you stay awake, and let people you trust curate your news a bit.

Organize your sources with automation tools. These are apps that consolidate your news consumption and information collecting by automating how you read it and save it for later. RSS readers will let you organize news sources you choose into useful lists and timelines in order of time posted—no interference by algorithms. And who doesn't love less notifications? Great RSS readers include Feedly, Inoreader, Feeder, Newsblur, Tiny Tiny RSS, Feedbin, and FreshRSS.

A bookmarking app will save anything for you to read later, like an article, thread, PDF, or link. You can also create folders to organize your topics. When you see an article you want to read, add it to the Instapaper folder according to its subject with one click, where it will be saved. Then read the article when you make time and have the spoons to process it. Some good bookmarking apps are Instapaper, Pocket, Raindrop.io, PaperSpan, Matter, Omnivore, Evernote, or Flipboard.

Regulate your intake. I try to remind myself that "drinking from the firehose will kill you."

Set a limit on your Covid scrolling hours and put them into a routine with breaks baked in. This way you have a time set aside to read the news and process any distress you may feel. Decide on a baseline of hours each day for you to spend on reading news and scrolling apps. This is your target. One Covid-conscious psychologist I consulted said, "I know that I personally was spending nearly four hours a day on news, and finally had to decide an hour was enough." Don't be hard on yourself about going over your target: it's a tool to mitigate the damage of overwhelm and it's okay to be flexible.

CONNECT WITH THE THINGS YOU CAN DO

We've seen our friends and loved ones, who might otherwise be smart and sensible about Covid-19 prevention, bafflingly decide to give up.

Much of what we're seeing is an overwhelming sense of futility. Despair is an alluring place to get stuck when your friends "don't want to hear the C-word" or your kids' daycare is full of children whose parents "just can't figure out why everyone is sick all the time." It's tempting to give in to hopelessness when there's no support for prevention from leadership.

Taking action feels impossible when showing up in person anywhere is high-risk, from indoor maskless meetings to mask-ban protests. For disabled and chronically ill people, including the exploding population of people with Long Covid, showing up in person, or even extended screen time is a decision made with a very low budget of baseline ability—for which a price will be paid later. And yet these are the very people who have been made to shoulder the burden of advocating for their own recognition, healthcare needs, prevention requirements, and for change.

When you start to feel like no one cares and changing our circumstances is impossible, or that you don't have enough time to be part of a solution, you have just one job: connect with the things you *can* do.

There are many ways we can accomplish magnitudes without needing to risk infection (or a Long Covid crash) in person, without having to carve out nonexistent spare time, or even having to squeeze out your last drops of optimism.

Share articles and prevention information. Articles you share don't necessarily need to be new: resurface any of journalist Ed Yong's Covid-19 coverage from *The Atlantic* on social media or send links to friends and family. Much of the latest prevention news never gets off social media: text or email articles about how awesome N95s are to potentially receptive recipients. If an essay by Alice Wong moves you, send it to someone who might not see it otherwise. See a headline asking why we have to keep getting Covid over and over again? Make sure one other person sees it, too. Small things add up: this includes likes.

Make one-time or recurring donations. There are many great causes that need our help right now, and even one teeny-tiny donation will help. If you can, consider setting a recurring donation so that you're always doing *something* even when you feel like you're not. Consider Long Covid Kids, The Corsi-Rosenthal Foundation, The Disability Visibility Project, or the Longhauler Advocacy Project. Visit the Covid Action Map to find over 100 mask blocs worldwide, advocacy organizations, clean air orgs, prevention events, and many more.

Sign online petitions. Trust me, even just one signature helps when you add your voice and presence to a group of people demanding change, attention for research, or showing politicians that prevention matters. In a recent Covid action meeting I virtually attended, one member recounted their conversation with a public health official about how soon the public could expect booster shot access. The official commented saying they didn't know if there was enough demand—signatures on petitions are one key way to show that.

Amplify accurate Covid-19 information and prevention resources. Come across a really easy to understand guide for clean air indoors? Share it: most people think air purifiers and CO_2 are "too complicated." They're not wrong! Did you find a mask discount, an online retailer having an N95 clearance sale, local Paxlovid access information, or air purifiers with free shipping? Someone you don't even know is looking for exactly that, and might come across your share. Share the Covid Action Map, the Clean Air Club, the Clean Air Crew, The John Snow Project, or The Sick Times.

Try microvolunteering. This is where you perform small, low-commitment tasks for organizations that need stuff done. Not all volunteering is a huge commitment, nor does it need to be done in person.

Find an organization you'd like to support and look for their volunteering information. The World Health Network "is open to anyone interested in curtailing the spread of COVID-19 and its harmful effects regardless of education or field of expertise." The "Volunteer with Clean Air Club" page presents 22 different options ranging from "alt-text writer" and "advocacy" to "other," with flexible choices for how much time you can spend.

Give emotional support to people fighting for change. A little goes a long way here: every single person doing the hard work of defying gaslighting and staring into the sun of Covid's realities is experiencing the trauma of bearing witness. Many have people they love who are suffering, or are fighting for their own lives just as much as for others. Your kind words can carve out a moment that tells someone their efforts are worth it, they are seen, and that they matter. Listening and validating someone's experience and feelings is nourishment for those who dare to speak up, dare to do.

ADVOCACY: BE AN ALLY

You may have heard the phrase "Hospitals are the safest place you can be." Nothing is further from the truth right now. Hospitals, treatment centers, and doctor's offices around the world have rolled back the clock on disease prevention with anti-masking policies and an institutional willingness to infect patients with Covid-19 through prevention avoidance and staff greenlit to minimize Covid. For groups already facing systemic healthcare discrimination—BIPOC, LGBTQIA+, disabled, and women—"Covid is over" messaging from leadership is akin to making a trip to the ER into a potential death sentence.

For these targeted groups, healthcare's collective Covid denial has been like dumping fuel on a fire when it comes to the gaslighting, derision, dismissal, denial of treatment, hostility, and disbelief they already faced when trying to get care from people who would rather we simply don't exist.

Being afraid of going to a doctor is a terrifying way to live. No one should have to fight for a doctor to believe them or face ignorant myths about pain tolerance. None of us should have to beg sneering nurses to wear a mask—and go ignored or be pathologized. No one should be getting infected with Covid-19 because they went to the hospital (also called Hospital Acquired Infections aka Nosocomial Infections). None of us should be losing friends and family members after hospital-acquired infections. Black people should never have to team up to take their individual cases to press outlets because doctors insist their Long Covid symptoms are in their head.

Enraging? Completely. Take that anger energy and funnel it into sharpening your advocacy knowledge and skills. First, make sure you have express, clear consent from the person you're advocating for before you try to advocate for them. Your intentions to help can backfire and end up jeopardizing someone's care and comfort if you and the person you're advocating for haven't agreed to your plans beforehand.

Next, get prepped and organized. In *How to be an Effective Advocate for a Disabled Patient,* The Disabled Ginger describes in detail how advocates can be more effective in healthcare settings.[14] It's specific to disabled and chronically ill people but is applicable to advocacy for people in groups targeted by medical gaslighting. In brief, Disabled Ginger explains:

• Learn everything you can about what's affecting the person you're advocating for

- Keep multiple copies of all documents with you
- Know their current medications and med schedule, and be aware of allergies or contraindications
- Make sure you both have a "go bag" in case it's a longer stay than you expect
- Bring something for comfort or entertainment; podcasts, games, tablet
- Connect with on-premises advocacy support: chaplain, social worker, patient relations
- Disabled Ginger wrote: "Wear a mask. It will also be much easier for you to convince healthcare workers to mask if you're leading by example and wearing a respirator. Consider bringing extra respirators to provide to staff and make sure they know that no one is to come in contact with the patient unless wearing a mask."

"Be firm and clear but careful not to cause additional conflict. Try and learn the signs that the patient may be experiencing gaslighting or being unfairly psychologized," Disabled Ginger advises. "Work on unlearning your own ableism... Many people don't even realize they've got internalized ableism but we ALL have it... Being an advocate or caregiver is incredibly hard work. It's often unpaid and can be a thankless job—but it's one of the most important things you can do for people with disabilities." Be sure to read The Disabled Ginger's five-part series on what disabled and chronically ill people face in medical settings and being an effective advocate.

REFERENCES AND RESOURCES

INTRODUCTION: STAND TOGETHER

REFERENCES

[1] The Beginnings of Global Health at UCSF (UCSF Institute for Global Health Sciences)

[2] When rumours derail a mass deworming exercise (Lancet, 2007)

[3] San Francisco Announces First Local Cases of Coronavirus (NBC Bay Area, 2020)

[4] Bay Area orders 'shelter in place,' only essential businesses open in 6 counties (The San Francisco Chronicle, 2020)

[5] SF COVID-19 response led to one of lowest death rates about U.S. cities, study finds (CBS News, 2023)

[6] On COVID-19, the United States Still Lags Behind Peer Countries (Think Global Health, 2023)

[7] The COVID Tracking Project (Reveal, 2023)

[8] The Worst Covid Strategy Was Not Picking One (Bloomberg, 2023)

[9] The best and worst places to be in the Coronavirus era (Bloomberg, 2020)

[10] Covid-19: Why NZ's life-saving elimination strategy didn't come with 'bounce-back' in deaths (Newstalk ZB, 2023)

[11] Minimising harms from COVID-19 and other respiratory infections (University of Otago, 2023)

CHAPTER 1: WHY WE STAY SAFE

REFERENCES

[1] Refrigerated trucks requested in Texas and Arizona as morgues fill up due to coronavirus deaths (Washington Post, 2020)

[2] NYC still storing COVID-19 victims in refrigerated trucks (AP, 2021)

[3] Health and Care Worker Deaths during COVID-19 (WHO, 2021)

[4] What is the impact of long-term COVID-19 on workers in healthcare settings? A rapid systematic review of current evidence (NIH, 2024)

[5] What's the Difference Between Shelter in Place, Safer at Home, and Stay Home Orders? (NLC, 2020)

[6] "FACT: #COVID19 is NOT airborne." (WHO, Twitter, March 28, 2020)

[7] Airborne transmission of SARS-CoV-2: The world should face the reality (Environment International, ScienceDirect, 2020)

[8] Whose breath are you breathing? (RNZ, 2022)

[9] The WHO overturned dogma on how airborne diseases spread. Will the CDC act on it? (NBC News, 2024)

[10] Protecting Against COVID-19 and Other Infections in Early Care and Education Programs (US CDC, 2024)

[11] Inside the Biden administration abrupt reversal on masks (Washington Post, 2021)

[12] The Millions of People Stuck in Pandemic Limbo (The Atlantic, 2022)

[13] Highlighting COVID-19 racial disparities can reduce support for safety precautions among White U.S. residents (NIH, 2022)

[14] An Incalculable Loss (The New York Times, 2020)

[15] U.S. Surpasses 1 Million Known Covid Deaths (The New York Times, 2022)

[16] The pandemic's true death toll (The Economist, 2022)

[17] Coronavirus Disease 2019 and Airborne Transmission: Science Rejected, Lives Lost. Can Society Do Better? (Oxford Academic, 2023)

[18] Evidence from whole genome sequencing of aerosol transmission of SARS-CoV-2 almost 5 hours after hospital room turnover (AJIC, 2024)

[19] Ambient carbon dioxide concentration correlates with SARS-CoV-2 aerostability and infection risk (Nature, 2024)

[20] Interim Guidelines for Biosafety and COVID-19 (US CDC, 2024)

[21] The Proportion of SARS-CoV-2 Infections That Are Asymptomatic : A Systematic Review (PubMed/NIH, 2021)

[22] Booster waning, Long Covid brain fog, and potential of Paxlovid resistance (Eric Tool/Ground Truths, 2022)

[23] More proof COVID is a multi-system cluster bomb (InSight, 2022)

[24] COVID and the Heart: It Spares No One (Johns Hopkins, 2022)

[25] Does COVID-19 damage the brain? (Harvard Health Publishing, 2023)

[26] COVID-19 and Immune Dysregulation, a Summary and Resource (World Health Network, 2023)

[27] Coronavirus Deranges the Immune System in Complex and Deadly Ways (KFF Health News, 2021)

[28] The Kids Were Safe From COVID the Whole Time (New York Magazine, 2021)

[29] Long COVID is a "public health crisis for kids," experts say (Salon)

[30] Study reveals majority of pediatric long COVID patients develop a dizziness known as orthostatic intolerance (MedicalXpress/Archive MD)

[31] Young children have a different immune response to COVID – Expert Reaction (Science Media Centre NZ, 2024)

[32] People with COVID Often Infect Their Pets (Scientific American, 2021)

[33] COVID infection can damage the brains of dogs, study suggests (CIDRAP, 2023)

[34] Nearly One in Five American Adults Who Have Had COVID-19 Still Have "Long COVID" (CDC, 2022)

[35] Half of COVID-19 patients report symptoms after 12 weeks, says new PHAC review (CTV, 2021)

[36] Long COVID: Lasting effects of COVID-19 (Mayo Clinic, 2024)

[37] Long COVID (Post-COVID Conditions, PCC) (Yale Medicine, 2024)

[38] Notice of Retraction: Hahn LM, et al. Post–COVID-19 Condition in Children (JAMA Pediatrics, 2024)

[39] Long COVID science, research and policy (Nature Medicine, 2024)

[40] Every COVID Infection Increases Your Risk of Long COVID, Study Warns (UNMC, 2023)

[41] What doctors wish patients knew about COVID-19 reinfection (AMA, 2023)

[42] What You Need to Know About Being Immunocompromised During COVID-19 (Penn Medicine, 2022)

[43] COVID-19 Cases and Deaths by Race/Ethnicity: Current Data and Changes Over Time (KFF, 2022)

[44] An intersectional analysis of long COVID prevalence (International Journal for Equity in Health, 2023)

[45] Long-COVID rate among disabled people double that of able-bodied (CIDRAP, 2024)

[46] Black, Hispanic people may be more likely to have long COVID but not be diagnosed (CIDRAP, 2023)

[47] KFF COVID-19 Vaccine Monitor September 2023 (KFF, 2023)

[46] Omicron BA.5 strain may shorten COVID immunity from 3 months to 28 days, research shows (ABC7, 2022)

[49] Half of Americans never think they'll get COVID again (Ipsos, 2024)

CHAPTER 2: TRUST THE TOOLS

REFERENCES

[1] Covid-19 and the Swiss cheese system (University of Auckland, 2022)

[2] The differences between masks and respirators (3M, 2020)

[3] Masks and respirators for prevention of respiratory infections: a state of the science review (Clinical Microbiology Reviews, 2024)

[4] Masks Work. Distorting Science to Dispute the Evidence Doesn't (Scientific American, 2023)

[5] Flo Mask (flomask.com)

[6] Mask Squad Cartel (masksquad.bigcartel.com)

[7] Steadirob (cults3d.com/en/users/steadirob/3d-models)

[8] Mask Nerd (YouTube)

[9] Fit Test the Planet (testtheplanet.org)

[10] MaskTogetherAmerica Mask Chart (MaskTogetherAmerica)

[11] Everything You Need to Know About Mask Braces: Do They Work? Can You Make Your Own? (Popular Mechanics, 2021)

ADDITIONAL MASK RESOURCES

Mask braces: Fix the Mask (fixthemask.com)

Reputable mask sources: Project N95, PPEO KN100s, Bonafide masks, DemeTECH, Family Masks, BE HEALTHY, MaskLab, Armbrust Mask Sampler Kit, Canada Strong, Envo Mask, ReadiMask, [breathe], CanadamasQ, black N95s, breatheTeq, Masklab Global

[12] Improving ventilation (Aotearoa Covid Action)

[13] How much natural ventilation rate can suppress COVID-19 transmission in occupancy zones? (National Library of Medicine/NIH, 2024)

[14] Busy mom builds a PC fan Corsi-Rosenthal box (It's Airbourne, 2023)

[15] DIY box fan filters – Corsi-Rosenthal box (Clean Air Crew)

[16] The Corsi-Rosenthal Foundation (corsirosenthalfoundation.org)

[17] A CFD study on the effect of portable air cleaner placement on airborne infection control in a classroom (Environmental Science, 2024)

[18] Portable HEPA Purifiers to Eliminate Airborne SARS-CoV-2: A Systematic Review (National Library of Medicine/NIH, 2022)

[19] Personal Portable Air Purifier Necklaces: Do They Work? (Smart Air, 2024)

[20] Far-UVC Light Can Virtually Eliminate Airborne Virus in an Occupied Room (Columbia University, 2024)

[21] Intro to Upper-Room UVGI (It's Airborne)

[22] Nukit 222 (nukit222.com)

[23] Virus lifespan and transmission boosted by high CO2 levels (Earth, 2024)

[24] Ambient carbon dioxide concentration correlates with SARS-CoV-2 aerostability and infection risk (Nature Communications, 2024); How Carbon Dioxide Increases a Virus's Lifetime in the Air (YouTube)

ADDITIONAL AIR RESOURCES

Covid and Other Respiratory Germs: No More Respiratory Infections (Air Support Project)

8+ Best Carbon Dioxide Monitors – What You Need to Know (Breathe Safe Air)

Aranet4 (aranet.com)

Simple things you can do to avoid COVID (Aranet)

In-Depth Lesson Videos, Air Quality (UC Davis College of Engineering)

How to build your own Corsi-Rosenthal Box (The Corsi-Rosenthal Foundation)

[25] COVID-19 vaccination may lower the risk for long COVID (Harvard Medical School, 2024)

[26] Booster waning, Long Covid brain fog, and potential of Paxlovid resistance (Eric Tool/Ground Truths, 2022)

[27] Are Rapid COVID-19 Test Results Reliable? (Healthline, 2022)

[28] Study Examines Performance of Serial COVID Testing (Northwestern Medicine, 2023)

[29] 15 things not to do when using a rapid antigen test, from storing in the freezer to sampling snot (The Conversation, 2022)

[30] How Long Are You Contagious With COVID-19? (GoodRx, 2024)

[31] Covid-19 Histamine theory: Why antihistamines should be incorporated as the basic component in Covid-19 management (NIH, 2024)

[32] Will COVID nasal sprays soon help prevent and treat infection? (NewsGP, 2022)

[33] Nasal sprays for treating COVID-19: a scientific note (Springer, 2023)

[34] Clinical efficacy of nitric oxide nasal spray (NONS) for the treatment of mild COVID-19 infection (NIH, 2021)

[35] SARS-CoV-2 accelerated clearance using a novel nitric oxide nasal spray (NONS) treatment: A randomized trial (Lancet, 2022)

[36] Iota-Carrageenan Inhibits Replication of the SARS-CoV-2 Variants of Concern Omicron BA.1, BA.2 and BA.5 (Nutraceuticals, 2023)

[37] Ethyl lauroyl arginine hydrochloride (ELAH) nasal spray as potent antiviral against SARS-CoV-2 (News-Medical, 2022)

[38] Intranasal Xylitol for the Treatment of COVID-19 in the Outpatient Setting: A Pilot Study (Cureus/NIH, 2022)

[39] Intranasal neomycin evokes broad-spectrum antiviral immunity in the upper respiratory tract (Immunology and Inflammation, 2024)

[40] Clinical Effects of Streptococcus salivarius K12 in Hospitalized COVID-19 Patients: Results of a Preliminary Study (Microorganisms/NIH, 2022)

[41] Oropharyngeal Probiotic ENT-K12 Prevents Respiratory Tract Infections Among Frontline Medical Staff Fighting Against COVID-19: A Pilot Study (Frontiers in Bioengineering and Biotechnology, 2021)

[42] Mouthwashes with CPC Reduce the Infectivity of SARS-CoV-2 Variants In Vitro (Journal of Dental Research/NIH, 2021)

[43] Oral mouthwashes for asymptomatic to mildly symptomatic adults with COVID-19 and salivary viral load: a randomized, placebo-controlled, open-label clinical trial (BMC Oral Health, 2024)

[44] Stoggles (stoggles.com)

[45] Sip Mask (sipmask.com)

CHAPTER 3: PLAN IT, JANET

REFERENCES

[1] Relative efficacy of masks and respirators as source control for viral aerosol shedding from people infected with SARS-CoV-2 (eBio Lancet, 2024)

[2] Is one-way masking enough? (Canadian Medical Association Journal, 2022)

[3] Scientists discover higher levels of CO2 increase survival of viruses in the air and transmission risk (University of Bristol, 2024)

[4] Evidence from whole genome sequencing of aerosol transmission of SARS-CoV-2 almost 5 hours after hospital room turnover (American Journal of Infection Control, 2024)

[5] Analysis of a super-transmission of SARS-CoV-2 omicron variant BA.5.2 in the outdoor night market (Frontiers in Public Health, 2023)

[6] The Risk of Aircraft-Acquired SARS-CoV-2 Transmission during Commercial Flights: A Systematic Review (International Journal of Environmental Research and Public Health, 2024)

[7] SARS-CoV-2 aerosol risk models for the Airplane Seating Assignment Problem (Journal of Air Transport Management, 2018)

[8] Behaviors, movements, and transmission of droplet-mediated respiratory diseases during transcontinental airline flights (Applied Biological Sciences, 2022)

[9] 13 Things To Know About Paxlovid (Yale Medicine, 2024)

[10] Metformin: Outpatient treatment of COVID-19 and incidence of post-COVID-19 condition over 10 months (Lancet Infectious Diseases, 2023)

[11] Should You Use a Pulse Ox When You Have COVID-19? (Healthline, 2022)

[12] Detailed study reveals how pulse oximeters significantly overestimate oxygen readings in people with darker skin tones (University of Plymouth, 2024)

[13] How Long Are You Contagious With COVID-19? (GoodRX, 2024)

[14] Why You Should Rest—a Lot—If You Have COVID-19 (TIME, 2022)

[15] How soon can I get COVID again? Experts now say 28 days – but you can protect yourself (The Conversation, 2022)

RESOURCES

Being safer in high-risk environments (Aotearoa Covid Action)

Safer In Person Gatherings Guide (People's CDC, 2023)

Postpartum: covid mitigations we took during labor (planned C Section) (California Codes/Threadreader, 2022)

What to Do When I Have Covid (Clean Air Club)

What to Do if You Have Covid (People's CDC, 2023)

What To Do If You Catch Covid (Roots Community Health Center video series, YouTube, 2023)

Someone in my home has COVID. How do we isolate safely? (Clean Air Crew)

What to do if you get covid (Monkeys on Typewriters, 2024)

CHAPTER 4: COVID BOUNDARIES

RESOURCES

10 Ways to Build and Preserve Better Boundaries (PsychCentral, 2021)

How to Set Healthy Boundaries With Anyone (Verywell Health, 2024)

Setting COVID Boundaries (Olivia Belknap Therapy, 2024)

Setting Your COVID-19 Boundaries: 7 Strategies to Effectively Communicate With Loved Ones (Northwestern Medicine, 2022)

What to do when loved ones don't take COVID seriously (Piedmont, 2020)

CHAPTER 5: TALKING ABOUT COVID

REFERENCES

[1] Dianna's Patreon (patreon.com/physicsgirl)

[2] Physics Girl LIVE with long Covid (YouTube, 2024); Physics Girl Livestream Notes and Q&A (Google Docs, 2024)

[3] How to Talk to Your Loved Ones About Covid (Covid Tips, 2024)

[4] Asking for Safer Precautions (World Health Network)

[5] How to Stay Covid Safe When in Hospital (Part Three: The Disabled Ginger, 2024)

[6] Conspiracy theory (Britannica, 2024)

[7] Bad News (disinformation media literacy game)

[8] Go Viral! (World Health Organization's Covid-19 misinformation literacy game)

[9] DebunkBot (debunkbot.com)

[10] DebunkBot | Some Dare Call It Conspiracy (somedarecallitconspiracy.com)

RESOURCES

Coronavirus disease (COVID-19) advice for the public: Mythbusters (World Health Organization, 2022)

We Need to Talk About Misinformation and Disinformation (Enthusiastic Encouragement & Dubious Advice, 2024)

You Have to Live Your Life (research responses to covid gaslighting phrases)

How to Talk to Friends & Family Who Share Misinformation (Los Angeles Public Library, 2020)

CHAPTER 6: COVID GASLIGHTING

REFERENCES

[1] COVID Hasn't Disappeared — But Empathy, Care and Solidarity Have (Truthout, 2023)

[2] Identifying Gaslighting: Signs, Examples, and Seeking Help (Newport Institute, 2024)

[3] Gaslighting (Psychology Today)

[4] Hundreds die of COVID after catching virus while in hospital (The Age, 2023)

[5] Disease detectives gathered at CDC event—a COVID outbreak erupted (Ars Technica, 2023)

[6] Systemic gaslighting of women with language (3Plus)

[7] Racial Justice Resources for Activists, Advocates & Allies (U Cincinnati)

[8] 'Abhorent': Disability Advocates Slam CDC Director for Comments on 'Encouraging' Covid Deaths (Rolling Stone, 2022)

[9] Why racism is a public health crisis (BBC, 2024)

[10] How to Recognize and Respond to Racial Gaslighting (Healthline, 2024)

[11] How 'Medical Gaslighting' Ignores Black Women With Long COVID (Word in Black, 2024)

[12] Love Me or I Shoot You (London Review of Books, 2024)

[13] Remarks by President Biden Celebrating Independence Day and Independence from COVID-19 (White House, 2021)

[14] As Recommendations for Isolation End, How Common is Long COVID? (KFF, 2024)

[15] Millions of US Children Experience Range of Long COVID Effects (JAMA, 2024)

[16] COVID-19 Cases and Deaths by Race/Ethnicity: Current Data and Changes Over Time (KFF, 2022)

[17] No 'Freedom Day'? UK could delay lifting of all Covid restrictions due to Delta variant (CNBC, 2021)

[18] A Positive Covid Milestone (New York Times, 2023)

[19] One in 5,000 (New York Times, 2021)

[20] Virginia's breakthrough case numbers are likely an undercount (Virginia Mercury, 2021)

[21] Remarks by President Biden on Fighting the COVID-19 Pandemic (White House, 2021)

[22] Press Briefing by White House COVID-19 Response Team and Public Health Officials (White House, 2021)

[23] Omicron Is Milder (New York Times, 2022)

[24] The Liberals Who Can't Quit Lockdown (The Atlantic, 2021)

[25] What's the Difference Between Shelter in Place, Safer at Home, and Stay Home Orders? (NLC, 2020)

[26] Did COVID Precautions Like Masking Actually Work? With David Leonhardt (Megyn Kelley, Facebook, 2022)

[27] The pandemic's true death toll (The Economist, 2022)

CHAPTER 7: LONG COVID AND RELATIONSHIPS

REFERENCES

[1] Infected in the first wave, they navigated long COVID without a roadmap (Reuters, 2023)

[2] How and why patients made Long Covid (Social Science & Medicine, 2021)

[3] Long COVID science, research and policy (Nature Medicine, 2024)

[4] COVID-19 reinfection ups risk of long COVID, new data show (CIDRAP, 2024)

[5] Long COVID (Post-COVID Conditions, PCC) (Yale Medicine, 2024)

[6] Long COVID: Lasting effects of COVID-19 (Mayo Clinic, 2024)

[7] Understanding ME/CFS and Long COVID as Post-Viral Conditions (Society to Improve Diagnosis in Medicine, 2022)

[8] Scientists are piecing together the puzzle of long COVID. Here's what to know (UNMC Global Center for Health Security, 2024)

[7] Denial Isn't an Effective Health Care Strategy, Say People With Long COVID (Truthout, 2023)

[9] Long COVID information-seeking experiences: Considerations to improve access to information and care (PIPPS, 2023)

[10] How You Can Support Loved Ones Living with Long-COVID (University of Colorado School of Medicine)

[11] What doctors wish patients knew about COVID-19 reinfection (AMA, 2023)

[12] People with long COVID continue to experience medical gaslighting more than 3 years into the pandemic (The Conversation, 2023)

[13] Understanding and Addressing Medical Gaslighting (Hodgkin's Blog, 2023)

[14] The long Covid nightmare is far from over, especially for women of color (PRISM, 2023)

[15] Long covid and medical gaslighting: Dismissal, delayed diagnosis, and deferred treatment (Elsevier/NIH, 2022)

[16] How COVID-19 Brought Medical Gaslighting to the Forefront and Made Invisible Illness Visible: Lessons from the BIPOC Long COVID Study. (COVID-19 Pandemic, Mental Health and Neuroscience - New Scenarios for Understanding and Treatment, 2022)

[17] We've only just begun to examine the racial disparities of long covid (MIT Technology Review, 2022)

[18] Long Covid: An Anthropological Perspective: Why Women Physicians (emilymendenhall.substack.com, 2024)

[19] Medicalizing disabled people's emotions—Symptom of a dis/ableist society (NIH, 2023)

[20] "But You Don't Look Sick": Medical Gaslighting and Disability Identity Among Individuals Living with POTS and ME/CFS (Bryn Mawr, 2021)

Medicalizing disabled people's emotions—Symptom of a dis/ableist society (NIH, 2023)

[21] Long haulers are redefining Covid-19 (The Atlantic, 2020)

[22] Psychiatric and neurological complications of long COVID (NIH, 2022)

[23] Fatigue Can Shatter a Person (The Atlantic, 2023)

[24] One of Long COVID's Worst Symptoms Is Also Its Most Misunderstood (The Atlantic, 2022)

[25] Neuropsychological Manifestations of Long COVID (Delaware Psychological Association)

[26] How health and safety are compromised for people living with long COVID and intimate partner violence (Lens, 2024)

RESOURCES

An Introduction to Long COVID for Mental Health Professionals (Delaware Psychological Association, 2024)

The Basics: Orthostatic Intolerance (OI) (Bateman Horne Center, YouTube, 2024)

The Basics: Post-Exertional Malaise (PEM) (Bateman Horne Center, YouTube, 2024)

The Bateman Home Center (Bateman Horne Center)

The Black Long Covid Experience (blacklongcovidexperience.com)

Co-Resting (co-resting.org)

COVID Recovery Center (US: Brigham and Women's Hospital)

Dysautonomia International (Dysautonomia International)

EEDA Newsletter Vol 5, Issue 5: How to Find a Therapist (Enthusiastic Encouragement & Dubious Advice, 2024)

The English National Opera Breathe Team (eno.org/breathe)

The Geek's Guide to Long Covid (guidetolongcovid.com)

Group Therapy with Clients with Long COVID (Delaware Psychological Association, 2024)

The Long Covid Action Project (linktr.ee/longcovidactionproject)

The Long Covid Alliance (longcovidalliance.org)

Long Covid Campaign (longcovidcampaign.org)

Long Covid Families (ongcovidfamilies.org)

The Long Covid Handbook (Linktree: all versions)

Long Covid Kids (longcovidkids.org)

Long Covid Justice (longcovidjustice.org)

Long Covid Learning (longcovidlearning.org)

Long Covid Moonshot (US) (longcovidmoonshot.com)

Long Covid Physio (longcovid.physio)

The Longhauler Advocacy Project (longhauler-advocacy.org)

ME Action (meaction.net)

Myalgic Encephalomyelitis/Chronic Fatigue Syndrome (ME/CFS) (Johns Hopkins Medicine)

Pacing and Management Guides (MEpedia)

Patient-Led Research Collaborative (patientresearchcovid19.com)

Pathogen Update: 9-5-2024 (Joseph Eastman)

Post-Exertional Malaise (MEpedia)

Postural Orthostatic Tachycardia Syndrome (POTS) (Dysautonomia International)

r/covidlonghaulers (Reddit)

The Sick Times (thesicktimes.org)

Survivor Corps (survivorcorps.com)

Why finding a therapist with a shared background has been my saving grace (Prism, 2024)

CHAPTER 8: COVID PERSONALITY CHANGES

REFERENCES

[1] Dark personality traits linked to health and safety risk taking, which can explain noncompliance with COVID-19 measures (PSYpost, 2022)

[2] Early Omicron Reports Say Illness May Be Less Severe (New York Times, 2021)

[3] Why Do They *Think* That? (Essays you didn't want to read, 2022)

[4] Why do People Stop Masking After They Get Covid…and How Should These Changes Inform Our Own? (Essays you didn't want to read, 2024)

[5] Can COVID-19 alter your personality? Here's what brain research shows. (National Geographic, 2022)

[6] 'The Rage Would Come Out of Nowhere': Personality Change Has Emerged as a Symptom of Long Covid (Rolling Stone)

[7] One of Long COVID's Worst Symptoms Is Also Its Most Misunderstood (The Atlantic, 2022)

[8] Post-COVID cognitive dysfunction: current status and research recommendations for high risk population (Lancet, 2023)

[9] Understanding the Impact of COVID-19 on Personality and Brain Function: A Grim Reality or a Wake-Up Call? (Infection Control Today, 2024)

[10] COVID-19 linked to long-lasting cognitive deficits, study finds (News-Medical, 2024)

[11] Sleep disorders of post-COVID-19 conditions (Springer: Sleep and Breathing Physiology and Disorders, 2023)

[12] The neurobiology of long COVID (CellPress Neuron, 2022)

[13] Short- and long-term neuropsychiatric outcomes in long COVID in South Korea and Japan (Nature Human Behavior, 2024)

[14] Neurocognitive and psychiatric symptoms following infection with COVID-19: Evidence from laboratory and population studies (ScienceDirect: Brain, Behavior, & Immunity - Health, 2022)

[15] Delay discounting: concepts and measures (APA PsychNet, 2012)

[16] COVID-19 and Traffic Accidents: Is a COVID-19 Personality Disorder Caused by Viral Damage to the Prefrontal Cortex? (Infection Control Today, 2022)

[17] Driving Under the Cognitive Influence of COVID-19: Exploring the Impact of Acute SARS-CoV-2 Infection on Road Safety (American Academy of Neurology, 2024)

RESOURCES

How to Use a Mood Tracker (Verywell Mind, 2023)

Best Mood Tracker Apps (Verywell Mind, 2023)

What is Impulsivity (Impulsive Behavior)? (WebMD, 2023)

ADHD Impulse Control: 5 Tips To Help You Manage (Psych Central, 2021)

21 Tools to Maximize Self-Control and Self-Regulation (Positive Psychology, 2020)

Volume 2, Issue 9: Adventures in Mental Health (Enthusiastic Encouragement & Dubious Advice, 2021)

What Is Habit Reversal Training? (The Recovery Village, 2023)

CHAPTER 9: ISOLATION AND CONNECTION

REFERENCES

[1] Out of control COVID means permanent segregation for many disabled people (The Gauntlet, 2024)

[2] Disabled People Have Unique Perspectives On Solitude (Forbes, 2020)

[3] Are You Socially Isolated? Learn the Signs and How to Get Support (Healthline, 2022)

[4] COVID-19 pandemic led to increase in loneliness around the world (APA, 2022)

[5] A Multi-Sectoral Platform Tackling Loneliness and Isolation Kicks Off (Japan NPO Center, 2022)

[6] Us vs. Them: The process of othering (Canadian Museum for Human Rights, 2020)

[7] Worldwide Mask Bloc Directory (maskbloc.org)

[8] Covid Meetups (covidmeetups.com)

[9] Covid Action Map (Google Maps)

RESOURCES

How to Reverse the Psychology of Othering (Psychology Today, 2023)

2024 BIPOC mental health toolkit download (Mental Health America)

Black Covid-19 Survivors Alliance (BCS Alliance; Facebook)

COVID Advocacy Groups Directory in US and Canada (Google Doc)

DIY long covid billboard toolkit (Google Drive)

Racial Justice Resources for Activists, Advocates & Allies [U Cincinnati]

The Disability Visibility Project (disabilityvisibilityproject.com)

Everywhere Accessible (everywhereaccessible.com)

r/Masks4All (Reddit)

r/COVIDgrief (Reddit)

r/COVID19_support (Reddit)

r/ZeroCovidCommunity (Reddit)

Pandemic Accountability Index (panaccindex.info)

The National Suicide Prevention Lifeline. Call the Lifeline at 800-273-8255, 24 hours a day, 7 days a week.

The Trevor Project. LGBTQIA+ and under 25? Call 866-488-7386, text START to 678678, or chat online 24/7.

Veterans Crisis Line: 800-273-8255, text 838255, or chat online 24/7.

Deaf Crisis Line: 321-800-DEAF (3323) or text HAND at 839863.

Befrienders Worldwide: International crisis helpline network to help you find a local helpline.

You are not alone (The Office for Policy on Loneliness and Isolation)

CHAPTER 10: MAKE ANGER USEFUL

REFERENCES

[1] The pandemic's true death toll (The Economist, 2022)

[2] Trauma (APA)

[3] How to stay in touch with our basic senses in isolation (CBC, 2020)

⁴ EEDA Newsletter Vol 5, Issue 5: How to Find a Therapist (Enthusiastic Encouragement & Dubious Advice, 2024)

⁵ Medicalizing disabled people's emotions—Symptom of a dis/ableist society (NIH, 2023)

⁶ Why Being Angry Is Okay (and Even Helpful) (Psychology Today, 2020)

⁷ The Final Pandemic Betrayal (The Atlantic, 2022)

⁸ National Covid Memorial Wall (UK: nationalcovidmemorialwall.org)

⁹ Marked by Covid: National Covid Memorial (US: markedbycovid.com)

¹⁰ COVID-19 Memorial Monument of Honor, Remembrance, & Resilience (Chicago: covidmemorialmonument.org)

¹¹ Grief Reaction and Prolonged Grief Disorder (NIH, 2023)

¹² What is Disenfranchised Grief? (HealthCentral, 2022)

¹³ All About Disenfranchised Grief (PsychCentral, 2021)

¹⁴ How to be an Effective Advocate for a Disabled Patient (Part Four: The Disabled Ginger, 2024)

RESOURCES

COVID-Conscious Therapist Directory (covidconscioustherapists.com)

Disenfranchised Grief (Sesame Street Workshop)

As a disabled person trying to 'live with' Covid in Australia, every day is a game of figuring out who is least likely to kill me (Guardian, 2022)

COVID-19 and Disenfranchised Grief (Frontiers in Psychiatry, 2021)

The Anxiety You're Feeling Might Be Pandemic Grief (TIME, 2024)

Disenfranchised grief (Taylor & Francis Online, 2009)

Emotional Analysis of Tweets About Clinically Extremely Vulnerable COVID-19 Groups (Cureus, 2022)

"I Won't Go to the ER Unless I'm Literally Dying." (Part One: The Disabled Ginger, 2024)

Tips for Surviving a Hospital Trip When Chronically Ill (Part Two: The Disabled Ginger, 2024)

How to Stay Covid Safe When in Hospital (Part Three: The Disabled Ginger, 2024, 2024)

How to be an Effective Advocate for a Disabled Patient (Part Four: The Disabled Ginger, 2024)

My Most Dangerous ER Experience and How My Advocate Saved My Life (Part Five: The Disabled Ginger, 2024)

Long Covid Kids (longcovidkids.org)

The Corsi-Rosenthal Foundation (corsirosenthalfoundation.org)

The Disability Visibility Project (disabilityvisibilityproject.com)

Longhauler Advocacy Project (longhauler-advocacy.org)

Covid Action Map (covidactionmap.org)

World Health Network (whn.global)

Clean Air Club (cleanairclub.org)

Clean Air Crew (cleanaircrew.org)

The John Snow Project (johnsnowproject.org)

The Sick Times (thesicktimes.org)

Rituals in the Making (ritualsinthemaking.com)

RSS readers: Feedly (feedly.com), Inoreader (inoreader.com), Feeder (feeder.co), Newsblur (newsblur.com), Tiny Tiny RSS (tt-rss.org), Feedbin (feedbin.com), FreshRSS (freshrss.org)

Bookmarking apps: Instapaper (instapaper.com), Pocket (getpocket.com), Raindrop.io, PaperSpan (paperspan.com), Matter (hq.g etmatter.com), Omnivore (omnivore.app), Evernote (evernote.com), Flipboard (about.flipboard.com)

BIBLIOGRAPHY

Blackstock, Uché. *Legacy: A Black Physician Reckons with Racism in Medicine* (Viking, 2024).

Diedrich, Lisa. *Illness Politics and Hashtag Activism* (University of Minnesota Press, 2024).

Douglas, Jon. *In it for the Long Haul: A Long Covid Journey* (Jon Douglas, 2024).

Duncan, Dustin T. and Kawachi, Ichiro and Morse, Stephen S. *The Social Epidemiology of the COVID-19 Pandemic* (Oxford University Press, 2024).

Easthope, Lucy. *When the Dust Settles: Stories of Love, Loss and Hope from an Expert in Disaster* (Hodder & Stoughton, 2022).

Garfield, Simon. *The End of Innocence: Britain in the Time of AIDS* (Faber, 1994).

Haines, Staci. *Healing Sex: A Mind-Body Approach to Healing Sexual Trauma* (Cleis Press, 2007).

Hassan, Shira. *Saving Our Own Lives: A Liberatory Practice of Harm Reduction* (Haymarket Books, 2022).

Hirsch, Lioba. *Antiblackness and Global Health: A Response to Ebola in the Colonial Wake* (Pluto Press, 2024).

Jackson, James C. *Clearing the Fog: From Surviving to Thriving with Long Covid—A Practical Guide (Little, Brown Spark, 2023).*

Kaufman, Miriam and Odette, Fran and Silverberg, Cory. *The Ultimate Guide to Sex and Disability* (Cleis Press, 2007).

Kenward, Louise. *Moving Mountains: Writing Nature through Illness and Disability* (Footnote Press, 2023).

Ladau, Emily. *Demystifying Disability: What to Know, What to Say, and How to be an Ally* (Ten Speed Press, 2021).

Ladd, Mary. *The Long Covid Reader: Writing and Poetry from 45 Long Haulers* (Long Hauler Publishing, 2023).

Law, Victoria. *Corridors of Contagion: How the Pandemic Exposed the Cruelties of Incarceration* (Haymarket Books, 2024).

Lewandowsky, Dr. Stephan and Cook, John. *The Conspiracy Theory Handbook* (Center for Climate Change Communication, George Mason University, 2020).

Lewis, Michael. *The Premonition: A Pandemic Story* (W. W. Norton & Company, 2021).

Linstrum, Erik. *Age of Emergency: Living with Violence at the End of the British Empire* (Oxford University Press, 2023).

Lowenstein, Fiona. *The Long COVID Survival Guide: How to Take Care of Yourself and What Comes Next* (The Experiment, 2022).

Medinger, Gez and Altmann, Danny. *The Long Covid Handbook* (Cornerstone Press, 2023).

Metzl, Jonathan M. *The Protest Psychosis: How Schizophrenia Became a Black Disease* (Beacon Press, 2021).

Newlevant, Hazel. *What's Up With COVID and How to Protect Yourself: 2024 Edition* (Hazel Newlevant, 2024).

Parish, Dana and Phillips, Steven. *Chronic: The Hidden Cause of the Autoimmune Epidemic and How to Get Healthy Again* (Houghton Mifflin Harcourt, 2021).

Prior, Ryan. *The Long Haul: How Long Covid Survivors Are Revolutionizing Health Care* (The MIT Press, 2024).

Ripley, Amanda. *The Unthinkable: Who Survives When Disaster Strikes—and Why* (Crown Archetype, 2008).

Samuel, Kim. *On Belonging: Finding Connection in an Age of Isolation* (Harry N. Abrams, 2022).

Schalk, Sami. *Black Disability Politics* (Duke University Press Books, 2022).

Shakespeare, Tom and Gillespie-Sells, Kath and Davies, Dominic. *The Sexual Politics of Disability* (Cassell, 1996).

Shilts, Randy. *And the Band Played On: Politics, People, and the AIDS Epidemic* (Stonewall Inn Editions, 1987).

Stephens, Morgan. *Tilt* (Kelsay Books, 2024).

Thrasher, Steven W. *The Viral Underclass: The Human Toll When Inequality and Disease Collide* (Celadon Books, 2022).

Weinberg, Kate. *There's Nothing Wrong with Her* (G.P. Putnam's Sons, 2024).

Wong, Alice. *Disability Intimacy: Essays on Love, Care, and Desire* (Vintage, 2024).

Wong, Alice. *Disability Visibility* (Vintage, 2020).

Wong, Alice. *Year of the Tiger: An Activist's Life* (Vintage, 2022).

Wright, Lawrence. *The Plague Year: America in the Time of Covid* (Knopf, 2020).

SURVEY RESPONSES

ON THE FOLLOWING PAGES you'll find anonymous results from *The Covid Safety Handbook* Survey, reproduced with permission. We've chosen a selection of responses for each question–it wasn't easy, there were hundreds! All of us in *The Covid Safety Handbook* community hope you find these helpful.

What's one thing you wish more people knew about Covid-19?

That they are not safe. That dismissing it as something only the disabled and elderly have to worry about is a lie, and they and their kids are at risk for disability with every single infection, no matter how young and healthy.

"Gateway drug" may or may not be a thing, but Covid-19 is indisputably the gateway illness to Long Covid.

Immunocompromised people had lives before this.

That they should still be planning their events with covid safety mitigations - ie venue air quality and masking.

It's airborne! Seriously, mainstream media is still talking about droplets and hand washing....

Anything at all! How to prevent, how to protect, how to survive it. People don't know anything and it's so frustrating we have to live like this.

It can affect you way after you stop testing positive.

Masking is far more important than cleaning surfaces.

It SHOULDN'T be an issue to want to protect yourself & loved ones. Anything else is weird.

That the pandemic is NOT over and that saying so only hurts people more (especially my immunocompromised friends who feel like shut-ins after 4 1/2 years).

I wish people understood how serious it is to get infected over and over. You can't keep subjecting your body to viruses in this way.

Avoiding infection isn't about not wanting to be sick for a week... It's about not wanting ticking time bombs in my body that result in worse outcomes for the rest of my life.

It can ruin your entire life in an instant, even if you are fit and healthy.

It's not mild or endemic; it's vicious.

Do you know someone with Long Covid?
Yes: 74.4%
No: 25.6%

What's one thing you wish more people knew about Long Covid?
That it can affect anyone, and it can destroy your life.

How likely they are to get it if they go around maskless.

If you become disabled with Long Covid, congrats, you're disabled now. There's no surefire cure, there's no guaranteed recovery, and there is no safety net.

People can look fine and still be very sick. People can have good days and bad days. It's often invisible, especially when you're just seeing someone for an hour or two.

That it's a real and actual thing currently without treatment or cure.

The person I know with long covid has been confined to bed for two years, unable to do any of the things she loved to do or to care for herself with 24/7 assistance. Taking the 5-10% risk that even a mild case of covid will result in this outcome is not worth, as Ed Yong phrases it, the "annihilation of possibility" from one's life.

That it's not just a long headache or a cold that won't dissipate, it's incapacitating. Societally, we're losing people down those cracks and they're losing homes, family, and ability to go on.

that it's not rare

I wish more people knew they were one small thing away from being disabled.

Powering through everything makes it more likely that you'll end up with long COVID, and powering through long COVID is a losing battle.

There aren't supports other than other disabled people.

Were you able bodied before long Covid? You aren't anymore!

Even if you've had covid before and were fine, you might not be so lucky next time.

I wish people knew that although it does attack the respiratory system, it isn't like other repository viruses because it infects cells in every major system and we are all left worse for the wear with every infection. So Long

Covid isn't about luck, it's just deadly statistics and how long you can roll safely on sketchy dice.

That it is a disabling illness striking down millions of people but entirely preventable.

Decline - especially cognitive - is not easily noticed. Your life will just get harder, in small or large ways, and you will be denied answers.

You never see those disabled by Long Covid, because they don't or can't get out. People drop out of public view one by one.

How do you feel when someone sets a Covid prevention boundary, like no indoor dining?

I love it.

It's me! I'm the one setting those boundaries, so when someone else does, I feel safer with them.

Great. Relieved. I have tons of my own Covid boundaries, and it makes me feel safer expressing them.

Elated - I can participate.

Supportive and ready to throw down as needed. I got infected in March of 2020 at work in fine dining, so it stung with particular detail to watch restaurants be a fulcrum of how the world refused to change.

Good (I am that person).

Extremely happy and grateful, because my partner and I have boundaries and covid protocols ourselves (we have a kink background.) They're structurally part of how we're navigating this together.

Great! Would make me feel a lot more comfortable and confident in doing things with that person.

Relieved that it's not just me setting boundaries

safe, hopeful

Empowered.

Great! Amazing! More of that, PLEASE!

Relieved! Happy! Seen! It's usually me setting the boundary and my friends (who all have looser risk profiles) kindly accommodating me.

When someone sets a Covid prevention boundary, like no indoor dining, I am hugely relieved to know that they care about their own and their loved ones health as much as I care about mine.

like they are someone who, as a disabled person, I can trust and would consider admitting to the small circle of people I actually spend time with anymore

Can we be friends???

What do you avoid because you don't want a Covid infection?
I avoid indoor dining and any indoor events.

Putting my kid in large crowds.

Any activity I cannot respie up during, including medical procedures. Indoor activities at all, outside my pod.

Crowds, and pretty much any public indoor anything.

Air travel, in-person healthcare, dating, hanging out with anyone unmasked

Going anywhere without my PPE/NPI satchel, plus prophylactic nasal spray, mouthwash, and antihistamine (loratadine).

So many things. Movies are a big one. I was a reviewer until 2016 and still saw 30ish movies a year pre-pandemic.

Theatre shows, gallery openings, parties, group dinners, Christmas with my family, the dentist (where I got my first infection)

Healthcare. Fun. Necessities. I'm a long hauler and it's so taxing. I want to wander and have fun like I used to.

When masking was higher, I mostly just avoided huge public events. But nowadays, no more dog parks, don't meet with friends or family often, don't bother meeting new people, any shopping in curbside or delivery, and almost entirely avoid food services now even if it's pick-up or delivery (haven't gone to a sit down place since pre-pandemic).

Healthcare where staff refuse to mask (or are happily unmasked) and refuse any accommodations.

Restaurants, cinemas, bars - nearly every place I went to regularly in 2019 (especially the ones that have closed permanently).

Everything; I limit family functions, I do the bulk of everything online, I have anxiety about going to the store, about what my kids will bring home from school, I don't go to concerts or movies or restaurants, bars or coffee shops anymore. People's unwillingness to take precautions to help everyone is killing me inside.

I was an avid concert goer, traveled a lot for roller derby, and I really miss karaoke. It's weird managing this and being single too. But I skip a lot now especially when the numbers are high.

Our church has moved to dipping the bread in the cup at Communion instead of sharing one cup between everyone and wiping it in between communicants.

Going to university and getting a degree, meeting other people without personal Covid measures, going to doctors, having a social life.

Most gatherings really. I got my second infection when gathering with family for my mothers celebration of life in June, I did not mask. Too difficult to deal with between peer pressure and grief.

Everything. I've barely left the house since March 2020. I just had a much-delayed, necessary surgery because I couldn't wait anymore. I've delayed so much important medical care, lost so many friends--all because I don't want to die from an avoidable illness.

Spending time playing tabletop games with friends. Going out to eat. Medical and veterinary appointments during surges unless critical.

What's a random Covid prevention tip you'd like to share?

Bring a small air purifier with you to work and any time you travel!

Wear a respie the same way you wear shoes - always in public, especially around people you don't live with.

Don't increase your risk because you haven't gotten it yet.

Masking saved my life. I was surrounded by my anaphylactic trigger and had no clue. I didn't even need my epi pen.

Assume that the germ is everywhere and act accordingly.

Make sure to be careful how you touch your mask when you take it off and then go wash your hands! If you were around anybody with covid, it's all over the outside of your hardworking mask.

To get a better fit out of flat-fold n95 masks, before putting it on, open the nose fold so it's completely flat. This will let it conform to your nose better and avoid a point that creates a gap.

Read the wind direction by turning your head until you can feel the wind in both ears.

Imagine each person you encounter is a campfire and you're trying to avoid their smoke.

If masks are uncomfortable, you likely just haven't found the right one yet!

Making an at-home fit test is easy and fairly affordable. It's also interesting and another layer in the Swiss cheese of protection.

Don't let hospital workers going unmasked give you a false sense of security.

Visualize cigarette smoke. Avoid situations where you would be breathing someone else's smoke.

Avoid people who refuse to mask the way you avoid sex partners who refuse to use condoms or safe words.

Anyone who doesn't respect your preventative choices doesn't deserve your respect.

Keeping lots of spare masks stashed in different places you frequent (home, office, car, etc) makes it easier to share masks if needed and to replace them when they break or get old.

Always look to see if there is a window that can be opened.

Keep your mask up, and wash your hands before you touch your face. If your nose itches, use a tissue not your fingers.

You will survive being the only person in a building wearing a mask. Sure, you probably won't make friends but you get to keep your health and live to fight another day.

Corsi rosenthal boxes can clean the air better than most filters, even ones much more expensive.

Minor gaps in masks can often be well sealed with double-sided clothing tape; if you just can't find one that fits perfectly, this may literally be a life-saver! (Note: leave tape on mask when removing, to prevent damage)

The best mask is the one that gets worn. So many people see this as an all-or-nothing fight, and it's not like that at all. If we can get more people to wear even cloth masks (I said what I said), we've made it safer for everyone.

As long as they're not crunched or bent or sweat damaged, N95 masks can just air out and keep being used week after week. Mount a hook by the front door and hang masks handy for door answering and going out.

If you have to remove your mask briefly for some reason be sure to first take a deep breath in with it on, hold your breath, remove your mask, put it back on, then exhale fully to push any possibly contaminated air out before breathing normally.

Not caring what other people think is a superpower.

I have a friend who is still masking and struggling with being alone. What do you want me to tell them?

You are not alone.

They are not alone. There are a lot of us out here. Get online. Find us. Look for hashtags like #YallMasking on places like tumblr. Join groups on Reddit or mastodon or wherever. It's on us to reach out and find each other.

There are lots of us. You may feel alone, but please know you are not alone. You're not crazy, or antisocial, or rude, or stubborn either. A tipping point will come, and we will find new ways to be in society and still keep one another safe.

Look for local advocacy groups. Consider getting on Twitter or Facebook. They're trash platforms, but they are also a really important tool for connecting with other Covid-safe people. For me, that's been key to ending feeling isolated.

There are still other folks out there willing to work within your boundaries. It's super hard to find out who, and awkward and troubling when someone won't, but I promise there are people who will if you ask.

Seek out support groups for solidarity, e.g. Mask Together America.

It fucking sucks, you are not alone.

They are seen and if we can help, we will. I do for my friends, but I came through the AIDS crisis, so this is for better or worse, not my first pandemic rodeo.

I would encourage the friend, to whatever degree their comfort level among others allows, upgrade that respiratory protection even further so they can trust it utterly. Specifically, decorated elastomerics kick ass. When you are ready, there is greater confidence to be found in accessorizing than trying to blend in with the mask-off world. To that end, and because of ocular ballistic droplet transmission, I also sincerely advise wearing louder sunglasses.

That there are ALWAYS more of us than they're going to see, in that so many of us cannot safely navigate the day to day right now.

There are a number of us who 'get it' and are fighting like hell day after day against the normalization of mass disabling. The gaslighting and peer/family pressure is tremendously thick, so finding support in whatever way you can to stay true to your own core self in relation to this is really important.

Hello fellow traveler, we have room for one more.

There's a poem "how to be alone" by tanya davis and filmed by andrea dorfman. It's on youtube. there's a line in it that sticks with me - "if you're happy in your head then solitude is blessed and alone is ok"

Can we be socially distant friends...?

It's worth it. Our healthcare system isn't built for taking care of people or healing really, to better to not catch what you can. I know it's hard, but no one else will love and protect you like you will. It's not okay. It's awful we got here. Grieving is a part of it.

Some of us are still in this together.

It's OK to feel exhausted with the struggle. Feeling the frustration, the exhaustion, the peer pressure, and choosing the right thing despite those feelings, is a spectacularly difficult form of adulting.

You're not alone! Even if you're the only one masking in your location right now, know that you have company somewhere. I'm often the only one masking in stores when I go out, and it's frustrating and it feels like I'm calling attention to myself in our politically conservative area, but I know that I'm doing it not just for myself but for all the people around me and for my family.

They are proving their solidarity, courage and steadfastness. There are many of us who are grateful and who stand with them. Kia kaha!

My kids sometimes struggle being (some of?) the only ones masking in their school. This summer we went to Pride, and even though they mostly stayed in the kids area, they still got some of the idea: they saw others wearing masks, and they said they felt less alone. I'm not sure this necessarily would work for others, but it warmed my heart. You're not alone: there are people taking care of themselves, their families, and their communities.

Any people who only accept you unmasked would never care for you in a worst-case situation. They want you for the good times, and would discard you for the bad.

you only get one body and it is important to protect it. disability (long covid) is just as isolating as avoiding covid. the gaslighting and invalidation and hostility you will receive when you get long covid will be just as bad as what you get for still taking covid seriously.

Your friend is not wrong because everyone is now ignoring Covid. The world is wrong for leaving us behind.

Your experience is so real. The situation has changed, including the social situation. Please keep seeking connection, whether individually on an app like Refresh or in groups on social media.

Find us; there's so many still coviding groups out there. We're on Facebook, we're in Discords, we're at libraries, masked, of course. You don't need to be alone.

Don't give up, it is worth it and there are other people who feel the same way and are willing to take precautions like masking, being outdoors, and testing (we use a Pluslife) to socialize in person, or if that's not possible doing remote hangs. Let's be friends!

You're not alone, you're not "imagining things" or "being paranoid." This is real, and it's hard, and I don't know when/if it'll get better, but giving up will absolutely make it worse. Find community where you can–there are people out there being just as cautious as you. Let's support each other, even if it's solely virtually because everyone in our physical lives has "moved on" from COVID. Let's survive this.

I'm so sorry our global public health systems have so drastically failed us to make this isolation necessary even after so long. I'm struggling too.

I think a lot of us are. Thank you for continuing to try to stay safe and slow the spread even as the wider world gives up. I'm grateful to hear that others haven't stopped taking this seriously.

You're not alone and you're worth it.

ACKNOWLEDGEMENT

THIS BOOK WAS ONLY possible because multiple communities that have formed or come together to prevent Covid-19, fight Covid gaslighting, restore community care, and reach out a hand when any of us have started to sink into despair showed up for this book, and sometimes for me, personally.

This book is in your eyes, hands, ears, and heart now thanks to the kindness, belief, and support of its 900 Kickstarter backers. I can't thank you enough for making a book we need so badly into a reality, and for being part of restoring community care along the way with your words, support, and validation of Covid prevention and all the hard decisions we have to make to stay safe.

The entire Covid Safety Handbook team wants to especially thank: Nicholas Slayton, Steven J. Vaughan-Nichols, Charles Lewis III, Davecat & Sidore, Gary and Nancy Goodenough, Antonia M., Gregg R., Kitty Stryker, Scott Squires, Chris Womack, Keith Hoodlet, Geoffrey Campbell, Richard Stringfellow, Jason Aller, Tina Hui, Bennett Elder, Cat Vincent, Kit Golan, Wil Broussard, Flavius S. Mercurius,

Ruth Sachter, Sarah Wolfe, em rodriguez, Philip Khor, Josefina & Luisa Topete, Maggie Konze, Tess B, Josh Simmons, Public Health Pledge, Sophie Luna, elkentaro, Rebecca Eichert, BEZA, acn128 & PriwallMoewe, Gregory G. Geiger, Maureen Batt, jennie douglass, The Haunted Bookshop of Iowa City, Steven Byrd, Alex Kell, Keri Kokke, Erika Rowland, C Gorzelnik, Sarah Cahill, Paco Hope, Jason 'XenoPhage' Frisvold, M. Yount, Alexander Dietrich, Matte and Cathy Edens, Elora Burns, Tara and Peter, Erica "Vulpinfox" Schmitt, Lee Worden, Victoria Wu, Allison Matthews, Julia Schiller, Thomas Rawls, Melanie & Jason, Zayvion Austin, Ryan De La Torre, Robin Kauffman, Ewen McNeill, Christopher Neal, Jaime Burnell, Joseph C, Dee Morgan, Paul Levinson, Dirk Karis, Khadija Hussain, Amanda Powter, Tamara J. Fingerlin, Elizabeth McCarthy, C. A. Bridges, Jessica Putnam Hughes, Calanish, Elizabeth Scheel-Keita, Codex O'Healey Melcher, Eugen Neuber, Antoinette Luzano, Fiona, OJ4HIRE, Stefan Kernjak, Jason Torrey McClain, Jon-Paul Dumont. David Turoff, Daniel Docherty, itgrrl, Sara Mitchell, Billy Smith, Andrew Hungerford, @chort@infosec.exchange, James Aylett, Kevin Schultz & Dawn Hustig-Schultz, Swiftdrawer, Peter Healy, David L Clements, Lauren Sabina Kneisly, Manuel Reichel, Jimmy Casas, Ginger Casas, Mia Casas, & Samuel Casas, Kricket Haberman, lilith, KariLikeSafari, Mylan Connolly, Nina Hatfield, mmalc Crawford, Frank Wales, Lauren Brennan, Meliarion, Claudine Chionh, J Gingras, Clifton Royston, Kai und der Andere.

This book also owes a debt of gratitude to the Stout Research Centre for New Zealand Studies and its research support for my forthcoming book about Aotearoa's Covid-19 response.

Thank you to Kira Omans for believing in this project, giving it a voice, and bringing the audiobook to life.

Thank you to my closest friend who stayed Covid safe with me all along, and never doubted me when I raised the alarm so many years ago: JWZ. Thank you to the friends who keep me strong: Richard Kadrey, Nicholas Slayton, Scotland Symons, KK, Thomas S. Roche, Ariel Waldman, Andrew and Megan, Kurt Collins, Patricia Elzie-Tuttle, Nicole Elzie-Tuttle, Anneke and Sean, Phillip + Limor + Luna, Geoff C., Vyrus, Eve Batey, Elizabeth, Ben Costa, Sean and Mila, Cecilia Tan, James Quilty, and Emerson.

Finally, I know they won't read this, but I wouldn't have made it through this book, the ongoing pandemic, or anything else without the loyal and loving companionship of the cats who take care of me in these isolating times: Max, who forever owns my heart, and Sam, a pandemic rescue who has made my "bubble" with Max into a cherished little family.

ABOUT THE AUTHOR

VIOLET BLUE (VIOLETBLUE.COM) IS a six-time Independent Publisher Book Award winning investigative journalist on cybersecurity, privacy, digital rights, and Covid-19, having bylined for *O The Oprah Magazine, Engadget, Financial Times, CNN, CBS News, The San Francisco Chronicle, Popular Science, The Spinoff*, and many others. *The Guardian* called Ms. Blue, "One of the leading figures in tech writing in the world."

Ms. Blue's books have sold over 2.2 million copies with translations in French, German, Italian, Spanish, and Russian. Her most notable book appearance was on *The Oprah Winfrey Show*. Her book *A Fish Has No Word For Water* won 2023 Independent Publisher Book Awards GOLD, was a National Indie Book Awards 2023 Finalist, a 2023 Kindle Book Awards Winner, and a Publishers Weekly BookLife Editor's Pick. BookLife/Publisher's Weekly described it as a "Superb memoir." KIRKUS called it "Gripping," urging readers to "Get it."

She is a member of the Internet Press Guild, The Authors Guild, The New Zealand Society of Authors, the International Federation of Journalists, PEN, the World Health Network, and Advisor to online legal privacy resource Without My Consent.

Ms. Blue has 15 years of experience in leading healthcare crisis communications workshops and trainings. This includes media trainings for UCSF Global Health Masters Program, Yearly UCSF Health immersive NGO trainings (Complex Humanitarian Emergency Training for Doctors Without Borders, American Red Cross applicants) and human rights conventions such as The Oslo Freedom Forum. Ms. Blue led trainings for San Francisco Sex Information's crisis workshops for nurses, therapists, and sexuality and gender students.

Her most notable charity contribution was donation of over 200,000 sales of *The Smart Girl's Guide to Privacy* to Médecins Sans Frontières/Doctors Without Borders, the International Rescue Committee, and the American Civil Liberties Union, raising £3.7m for migrant charities.

Ms. Blue's forthcoming book examines Aotearoa New Zealand's internationally praised Covid-19 response, with support from The Stout Research Centre for New Zealand Studies, Victoria University of Wellington.

www.ingramcontent.com/pod-product-compliance
Lightning Source LLC
Chambersburg PA
CBHW010329030426
42337CB00025B/4873